Breastfeeding

Empowering parents

Table of Contents

6

9

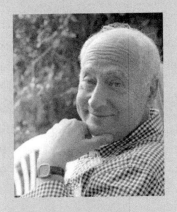

INTRODUCTION

Why this book? Do we really need another book on breastfeeding?

Yes, absolutely, the information in this book needs to be spread to parents, to health providers and in particular to physicians and pediatricians, hospital staff and lactation consultants. The lack of knowledge and understanding about breastfeeding amongst many people and, with a few exceptions, health professionals is dramatic, disheartening and devastating to so very many new mothers' and babies' experience with breastfeeding. So many mothers who were initially determined to breastfeed suffer excruciating pain. So many parents who were looking forward to their babies being breastfed are made to worry their breastfed babies are starving. So many parents are told by apparently rational health professionals that breastfeeding is not better than formula. So many parents are convinced, wrongly, that their baby has colic, or allergy to breastmilk or the baby is suffering "reflux" when, in fact, the issue is usually a breastfeeding problem which could have been prevented and can be treated, if only, if only the health provider knew what was really happening and knew what to do.

The lack of training of health professionals with regard to breastfeeding is shocking. Amongst pediatricians, who *should* know something about infant feeding, it is also disheartening. But pediatricians receive most of their "knowledge" about breastfeeding during their training. This means almost nothing of practical use. This means "there is a formula that is just right for every feeding problem".

And they also "learn" from their own or their spouse's experiences with breastfeeding which are frequently negative. When it comes to their own baby, they are completely at sea and surprised by the difficulties they encounter, and suddenly realize that nobody can help them. So, they turn away from breastfeeding and from then on "help mothers" who want to breastfeed by saying "my babies were not breastfed" and they are healthy and happy.

us not forget the "learning" they receive from formula company
,entatives who give them the latest on the "new and improved formulas,
.ch are almost like breastmilk and are the answer to almost all feeding
,roblems".

What do pediatricians learn in their training? I would suspect that at most universities, they learn much the same as they do at my own alma mater. I have seen the power point presentation accompanying the 1 hour lecture given to first year medical students. The power point is dated 2018, contains 44 slides, 4 of them concerning breastfeeding, all four of the slides giving dubious or frankly incorrect information about breastfeeding. These 4 slides are followed by 40 slides on formula feeding, most of them giving incorrect information. The basic message? There is a formula for every breastfeeding problem. Nothing, zero, zilch on preventing breastfeeding problems; nothing at all on how to help mothers and babies with problems.

It doesn't get any better once the student has graduated. After all, misinformation about breastfeeding is inherited from one generation to the next, located on the "formula information gene" or FIG and this gene is definitely dominant, passing from generation to generation from the 19th century and even before. The older pediatrician "teaches" the younger pediatrician, who teaches the resident in pediatrics who teaches the intern who teaches the medical student. And what do they teach? The same old, same old: lip-service to the badly formulated slogan of "breast is best", while at the same time stating frankly that the solution and certainty lie in formula which is not significantly different from breastmilk. And "please don't make mothers feel guilty for not breastfeeding". End of teaching.

After medical school and postgraduate training, virtually no learning about breastfeeding. Only "helpful" information from the formula company rep and formula company advertising. If the physician attends pediatric conferences, she or he will find not a single useful session on breastfeeding. But every formula company will have a booth in the vendors' area where well prepared representatives will inform the physician of all the improvements, high tech scientific changes to formula that have been made in the last few years.

So how did *I*, Dr Jack Newman, learn about breastfeeding?

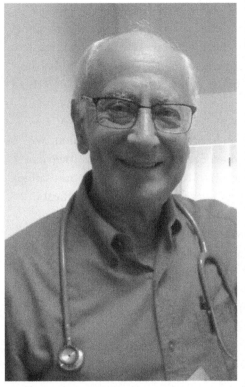

In 1983, I returned from working as a pediatrician in the Transkei, in Southern Africa. There, I saw that babies truly do die if they are not breastfed. I learned a little about breastfeeding, but I could have learned much more. I saw how the nurses in the pediatric ward could help a mother restart breastfeeding her starving child.

Why were the babies starving? Because the mothers were convinced that formula was best. White women mostly did not breastfeed, or if they did, they supplemented breastfeeding with formula. And White babies almost never died, unlike Black African babies who died frequently. The parents did not realize that the single most important reason that their babies died was the combination of formula feeding with *poverty* and that the reason White babies did not usually die was affluence, affluence, I might add, based on the backs of the Black African population.

Poverty was made worse by formula feeding, since formula was expensive, cost money that most Black African mothers did not have. As a result, they diluted the formula, often with contaminated water (all that was easily available). Most mothers could not afford to boil the water because firewood was also extremely expensive. Suffice it to say, it was a tragedy of enormous proportions.

When I returned to Canada, I worked as a staff pediatrician at the emergency department of the Hospital for Sick Children in Toronto. And in that role, I would see mothers who were trying to breastfeed their babies and were unsuccessful. Why? Because of a poor start with breastfeeding and poor advice from health professionals which often finished off the breastfeeding completely.

Thinking I could do better under different circumstances, since the emergency department was hardly the ideal place to help with breastfeeding, I suggested that the hospital could open a breastfeeding clinic. And against all odds, the idea was accepted. In the first full year of the clinic, 1985, we saw 70 mothers and babies.

Our breastfeeding clinic in Toronto now is located outside any hospital. We now see almost 70 mothers and their babies every week. We call ourselves the International Breastfeeding Centre. In addition to helping mothers and babies, we do research and we have students learning to be lactation consultants.

We have learned together over the years, and we have learned so very much. This learning came from listening to mothers, of watching the mothers breastfeed their babies, something that few physicians do. Most physicians will base the adequacy of breastfeeding on the baby's weight gain, a very poor way of knowing if breastfeeding is going well or not.

I had always thought that the goal of my clinic would be to make itself obsolete. Well, that obviously hasn't happened. If anything, the breastfeeding situation is worse now than it ever was.

Here are just a very few examples of the truly absurd things **I have heard from breastfeeding mothers:**

1. "My doctor told me that I should wear only white brassieres. Black ones will dry up your milk." From other sources, I hear that this piece of nonsense is not as rarely given to new mothers as one would imagine. I have no comment. There is no way to discuss this absurdity.

2. "If you breastfeed your baby, the antibodies in your milk will prevent the baby from developing his own immunity."

14

Comment: How absurd is that? If a baby is protected from developing infections by breastfeeding, that does not prevent him from being *exposed* to bacteria or viruses and developing his own immunity. The mother's antibodies and other immune factors in the milk help prevent the baby from getting sick, or, result in the baby becoming less sick than he would have been had he not been breastfeeding. But the baby still mounts his own immune response to the microbes (germs). In fact, this manner of being exposed to pathogens, with help from breastfeeding, is the best possible way of developing immunity.

3. "You should feed the baby only 5 minutes (choose any number) on each side and put the baby to the breast only every 4 hours."

Comment: Too many doctors, too used to bottle feeding, think that breastfeeding is like bottle feeding – just another method of delivering milk to the baby's stomach. Breastfeeding is not like bottle feeding, not the same even if the baby is receiving breastmilk in the bottle.

Part of the problem is that so many health professionals, and parents, have not been shown that a baby is not necessarily getting milk from the breast just because he has the breast in his mouth and makes sucking movements. It is for this reason that many mothers are told that their baby is not gaining well because the milk is "weak" or that the baby is getting only "skimmed" milk.

Setting time limits and intervals on how long and how frequently a baby should be at the breast is derived from "scientific" bottle feeding which used to happen routinely in the hospital setting (and is still very common even today) and was and is governed by hospital routines and not by the needs of babies who do not breastfeed solely in order to fill their stomachs with milk.

4. "My doctor says that formula feeding is better than breastfeeding, it is more scientific and safer for the baby." Clearly this is not true.

5. "I am taking an antibiotic for a throat infection and the doctor says I cannot breastfeed with this medication since it gets into the milk. But I don't understand. The baby is taking the same antibiotic." The vast majority of drugs do not require a mother to interrupt breastfeeding.

And we could go on for page after page after page.

So why this book?

In the hope that maybe, just maybe, doctors will read it and learn something. But more importantly, that parents learn a lot that will help them stand up to the incorrect, often absurd, comments and advice from health professionals. Because most mothers will read the information in this book and realize that it is correct, that it makes sense, that it is what they realized themselves. Maybe gift a copy of this book to your doctor or pediatrician.

BOOK AN APPOINTMENT AT THE NEWMAN BREASTFEEDING CLINIC

How to use this book

This book can be used in at least two ways. Some who want to use it as a textbook of breastfeeding may wish to read through it from page 1 to the end. But others may want to read different chapters at different times. For example, a pregnant woman awaiting her first child might want to start with how the practices around the labour and birth may affect breastfeeding success. A breastfeeding mother may want to look at the chapters about what is a good latch and why mothers may get sore nipples.

Each chapter stands on its own. If the information for the chapter for "what is a good latch" is important, as it is in many chapters, the link for it might appear several times on the same page. The idea is to have this extra information easily at hand for the reader and the reader not needing to search through the text.

Several chapters have information repeated, almost the same in each chapter. Again, this has been done so that the information is easily at hand, especially for the reader who is interested only one topic and wants easy access to extra information.

It is impossible to cover every single aspect of breastfeeding. We do not discuss breastfeeding of multiples, for example, because, though the logistics of breastfeeding multiples can be complicated, the basics of breastfeeding one or two or three are essentially the same.

THE RIGHT TO BREASTFEED

Many women who would like to breastfeed are not given the right to breastfeed their baby or the right to continue breastfeeding their baby. In fact, many mothers are being told that there is no difference between breastfeeding and artificial feeding and thus are not being given the information to make an informed choice about how to feed their baby. What woman would choose formula feeding if she were told that there is considerable evidence that mothers who breastfeed have a lower incidence of many serious diseases, including breast cancer, ovarian cancer and possibly uterine cancer, diabetes type 2 and that the longer she breastfeeds the lower her risk?

Are we kidding? Who is going to stop a mother from breastfeeding?

The truth

The truth is that mothers do not seem to have the right to breastfeed and are forced, by health professionals, by judges and by child protective agencies not to breastfeed from the very earliest days after the birth of their baby. And many are forced to stop breastfeeding if they have started.

Even when things are going well, mothers are frequently told they must add cow's milk to the baby's diet, presumably because "there is nothing in breastmilk after a year". They are often told they must stop breastfeeding altogether for this very reason, or because their child will be "overdependent" or incredible as it may sound, because breastfeeding past a certain age is abuse. This is not commonly said openly, but one child psychiatrist in France did make this statement to a widely read Belgian newspaper: "One does not share the breast: to extend breastfeeding past 7 months is without doubt sexual abuse". He is still much sought after by the media for advice on infant psychiatry. The mind boggles.

Mothers who had wanted to breastfeed and had trusted the health care system to help them prevent problems with breastfeeding or overcome problems with breastfeeding, are frequently left feeling guilty for not breastfeeding, feeling that they "failed" or feeling that they "couldn't" breastfeed for medical reasons. They

18

do not know that the health system actually undermined their breastfeeding and so, they blame themselves, not the hospital practices around labour and birth and after the baby was born and that undermined their breastfeeding. A lot of formula feeding by mothers who had originally intended to breastfeed would never have been "necessary" had the mothers been given the correct and supportive information and help that their medical condition or use of medication had not "required" them to stop breastfeeding.

The Fear of Starving the Baby

In addition, the parents' fear of the baby's health being compromised, or the baby starving, or suffering brain damage, are used as scare tactics to get mothers to consent to formula feeding and to shake their resolve to breastfeed. If doctors, nurses or dietitians actually knew how to know a baby is well latched on and how to know a baby is getting milk from the breast even in the first few days after birth, then the health provider would know if the breastfeeding is going well or not and would know how to help the mother and baby. And, if the breastfeeding is not going well, the health provider would be able to help the mother fix things *before* the baby gets into trouble. Because babies *do* get milk in the first days, *even with the first latch*, as shown by the pause in the chin as the baby opens to the maximum. The pauses are rather short *but present*. See a video on www.ibconline.ca showing a baby receiving milk from the breast. This baby is 3 weeks old, and the pauses are much longer than one would generally see on day 1 of life, but even on day 1, the pause should be present, indicating the baby is receiving milk.

Go to *www.ibconline.ca* to watch videos showing babies drinking from the breast or not.

What do Medical Doctors Know about Breastfeeding?

As a group? Though there are exceptions, doctors' knowledge of breastfeeding is so poor that if the slightest breastfeeding problem arises, the first thing many mothers will hear from the majority of doctors is "give the baby formula" or even "stop breastfeeding altogether". Mothers are often forced to supplement, or to stop breastfeeding completely, not infrequently in cases of slow weight gain, with the threat of the child protection services taking away the baby if they don't comply with "doctor's orders". This is appalling because the doctors who would do this, without referring to someone expert in management of breastfeeding problems, often haven't the slightest notion of what is going on and what can be done to improve the situation. They depend *only* on the baby's weight. And weights can be unreliable as a way of evaluating the adequacy of breastfeeding.

It is clear from our experience with many thousands of mothers having come to our breastfeeding clinic during the past 34 years, that much can be done to help the mother and her baby who is not gaining weight satisfactorily. With a little good help, the mother could carry on breastfeeding exclusively. However, in only a small minority of cases do the mothers actually get the help they need because the mother and baby are not referred to someone who *can* help. But that someone who can help is not usually the pediatrician, who should know, but only rarely does.

Sometimes the solution is easy. The way the baby is latching on can be adjusted so that the mother no longer has sore nipples and the baby gets more milk from the breast with this adjustment of the latch.

Another way of adjusting, or improving the latch is by releasing a baby's **tongue tie**. Sometimes the effect of releasing the tongue tie is dramatic in increasing the baby's intake of breastmilk, especially if the tongue tie is released early, in the first few days, before milk supply starts to decrease as a result of the tongue tie. A further method that can be used is **breast compression** which will increase the baby's intake of milk enough so that the baby does not need supplemental milk.

True enough, sometimes it's not so easy. However, even if breastfeeding needs to be supplemented, the supplements can be given with a lactation aid at the breast. This approach preserves the breastfeeding whereas supplementing with a bottle, the usual way recommended by health professionals, very often ends up with the baby refusing the breast and not breastfeeding at all.

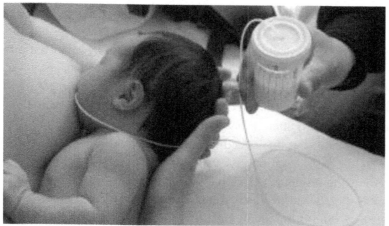

Using a lactation aid at the breast to supplement a baby when the baby may not be getting enough from the breast and other approaches to help the baby get more milk from the breast have not worked. Breastfeeding is not just about breastmilk. It is a relationship, a close, intimate, physical as well as emotional relationship between two people who are in love.

Unfortunately, most mothers do not get such help. Most of the time, mothers are left feeling frustrated and even devastated because they had desired to breastfeed and, due to the lack of qualified help or incorrect medical advice, they begin to see breastfeeding as "unreliable," necessarily "painful", "potentially dangerous" and ultimately, the importance of breastfeeding as "exaggerated". When women are prevented from breastfeeding when they had wanted to, they may become angry and traumatized, unable to see and experience the pleasure and joy of breastfeeding. Many resort to all sorts of coping mechanisms which resurface in discussions of infant feeding. One of the coping mechanisms is blaming breastfeeding, when it is not the fault of breastfeeding, but rather the fault of the system that let them down.

Below are just a few examples of how we take away mothers' right to breastfeed their babies. They highlight how society in general thinks about breastfeeding, how formula feeding is considered the standard way of feeding, and how breastfeeding is seen as a dispensable; nice, but not necessary.

What Information about Breastfeeding do Mothers Usually Receive?

Many obstetricians and family doctors will offer formula company "information" pamphlets, even beautifully done videos and not uncommonly will also give out formula samples to the pregnant woman, both "gifts" coming in a pretty, cute little bag, along with coupons to buy formula at a lower price. The "information pamphlets" (see photos below) often imply that formula is as good as, if not better than breastmilk and that breastfeeding is necessarily tiring and painful.

In fact, breastfeeding should not hurt. Nipples should not hurt; breasts should not hurt. If breastfeeding does hurt, something is wrong. The mother needs help, *good, hands on help.* But too many health professionals believe that pain is a normal part of breastfeeding and too often just advise mothers to "suck it up". These pamphlets tell mothers that breastfeeding is tiring, anxiety producing and furthermore, they strongly suggest that formula is a normal part of infant feeding, even if the mother and baby are breastfeeding just fine. The formula pamphlets and videos push the use of formula by saying it will allow the father to take part in the feeding of the baby and that, well, "sometimes, you just want to take a break", implying, of course, that breastfeeding is unpleasant and hard work. *It shouldn't be hard work.* In fact, mothers for whom breastfeeding is working well, will usually say how relaxing and easy breastfeeding is. But when breastfeeding is hard, it's because of how we help, or rather, don't help, indeed undermine, mothers' ability to breastfeed.

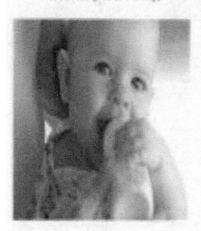

Typical, exploiting mothers' concern about their baby getting enough milk, and the solution? Formula, well, "our" formula, not another company's formula.

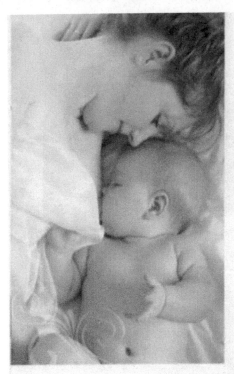

Feeding Problems Fixed

The smart Mom's guide to calming fussiness, spit up, colic and other common feeding challenges

By Deborah Swaney

When you're pregnant, the thought of feeding your baby conjures up all kinds of sunny, snuggly images. Then your child arrives, and faster than you can say "burp cloth," messy reality sets in. Newborns can have plenty of feeding-related problems—including gas, spit up, or colic—but fortunately there are simple ways to curb these.

Fussiness

What causes it? Overeating or swallowing too much air during feeding. **Signs to look for:** Fussing, either during or shortly after a meal. **What can you do?** Lots! For starters, if your baby is bottle feeding, try switching to a different nipple. "Artificial nipples are less supple than the real thing, making it harder for baby's mouth to form an airtight seal around them," explains Bridget Swinney, RD, author of Baby Bites: Everything You Need to Know About Feeding Babies and Toddlers in One Handy Book (Meadowbrook Press, 2007). "As a result, your baby may gulp air along with his formula, which gets trapped in his belly and causes discomfort." The solution? Experiment with different nipples until you find one that baby really latches onto.

Another strategy (for both nursing and bottle feeding Moms) is to feed your baby at the first signs of hunger. (Cues can include baby smacking his lips, opening and closing his mouth, or sucking on his hands.) "If you wait until he starts crying before you feed him, he'll swallow even more air as he starts drinking because he's so hungry," says Swinney. Feeding your baby when he's not so ravenous will result in a more relaxed, fuss-free experience.

*Of course, discuss feeding **problems** with a photo of a baby breastfeeding from a mother in a very awkward and likely painful position.*

24

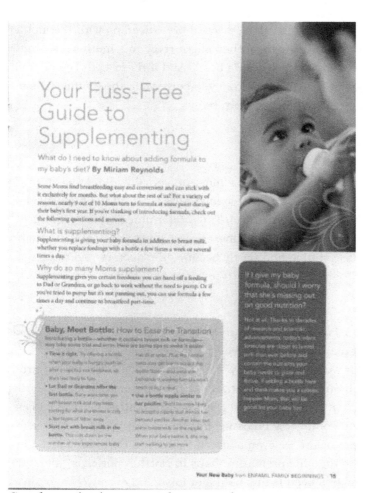

Supplementing is presented as normal, no problem, "fuss free". "Baby meet Bottle": Very cute. Bottle feeding is good and inevitable.

The above photos from a typical "information booklet" from a formula company tell the story. It is screamingly obvious that the "gifts" are meant to undermine breastfeeding. This is patently clear to the most casual of observers. When these "gifts" come from a person of authority like the family doctor or obstetrician, it means a lot. It's an endorsement of a product by someone the pregnant woman trusts enough to care for her and her unborn baby.

But do doctors, including obstetricians, discuss breastfeeding with the mother to be? With a few exceptions, the most they might reply to a mother's saying she plans to breastfeed is "good, breast is best". And if these "gifts" come from a family doctor or pediatrician after the baby is born, well, the mother trusts these people with the care of her now born baby.

Premature Babies

Mothers of babies born prematurely are almost universally told (at least in North America) that they cannot put the baby to breast until the baby is 34 weeks gestation (still 6 weeks premature). This undermines breastfeeding, partly because the baby could usually have started going to the breast much earlier than 34 weeks gestation and partly because the doctors and nurses frequently insist the "babies must to learn to bottle feed before they can breastfeed". Really?

Where does the idea arise that babies can learn to breastfeed by bottle feeding? And where does that magical age of 34 weeks come from? Not from any scientific studies. But we do know from work in Scandinavia that premature babies will often latch on to the breast at 28 weeks and sometimes even earlier than that. Not all, but at least some. And it is not rare that premature babies can be exclusively and completely breastfed (at the breast) by 32 to 33 weeks gestation, 1 to 2 weeks before we even allow the babies to try to breastfeed in North America. By the time the premature baby in North America is "allowed" to go to the breast, he has been fed by bottle for days and even weeks, often making initiating breastfeeding difficult. (It is necessary to add "(at the breast)" because so many in Western societies believe that giving breast milk in the bottle is breastfeeding – no, it's not at all the same).

Mothers of premature or sick babies or babies who are not gaining well are told that they must supplement with a bottle because breastfeeding is more tiring than bottle feeding. This false idea comes from the mistaken notion that babies have to work hard to get the milk out of the breast, that they suck milk out of the breast. But that is not how breastfeeding works. It is the mother who transfers the milk to the baby. The baby, of course, does his part, by

26

stimulating the breast to "release the milk". It is complete nonsense to say that breastfeeding is tiring for a baby, but it is widely believed, because most health professionals learn almost nothing about breastfeeding in their training and nothing at all after they finish their training. Most cannot tell when a baby is drinking milk from the breast and when the baby is *not* drinking milk from the breast. A baby is not getting milk from the breast simply because the baby has the breast in his mouth and making sucking movements.

Babies respond to milk flow (see video on www.ibconline.ca) and if the flow is slow, the baby tends to fall asleep at the breast, especially in the first few weeks of life. The baby falling asleep at the breast and then obviously still hungry after coming off the breast is taken as proof that breastfeeding tires out the baby. And this situation occurs simply because most mothers and most health professionals are not taught even the *basics* of breastfeeding, (including how to get a good latch, and how to know a baby is getting milk from the breast or not getting enough from the breast or something in between). Watch a video on www.ibconline.ca showing a baby born prematurely at 35 weeks gestation, but now at term, responding to flow from the breast.

Furthermore, breastfeeding has to compete with the flow the baby was receiving from the bottle and also the fact that the mother's milk supply is dwindling because the mother was pumping instead of being skin to skin with her baby and breastfeeding.

Babies do not tire at the breast. Babies respond to milk flow. It is a complete misunderstanding of breastfeeding to suggest that babies "pull milk out of the breast".

Mothers of babies born prematurely are almost universally told that their milk is not good enough for a premature baby and that the baby must receive "fortifiers", called "human milk fortifiers" which gives the *false* impression that the "fortifiers" are made from human milk. This is not the case (though "fortifiers" have been made from human milk). The "fortifiers" are actually made from cow's milk. Yes, sometimes "fortifiers" are helpful to make the baby gain more weight and assure adequate intake of nutrients, but in many NICUs (neonatal intensive care units) the use of "fortifiers" is *routine*! Even babies only a few weeks premature will receive fortifiers in many North American and European hospitals. But most of the time the "fortifiers" are unnecessary.

Some neonatologists or pediatricians will tell the parents that the baby needs to have breastmilk "fortified" until the baby is 10 months old. That is completely absurd. This is yet more work for the mother since to "fortify" the breastmilk, the mother needs to express her milk and add the "fortifier" to the expressed milk. And of course, mothers are giving this "fortified" breastmilk by bottle, which continues to undermine the breastfeeding. As a result, the truth is that most premature babies in North America leave the hospital bottle feeding. And. the parents leave the NICU believing bottle feeding was inevitable.

Babies at Risk for Low Blood Sugar

Mothers of babies born at risk for low blood sugar are often forced to give or allow the baby to be given formula (by bottle of course). But it is known that breast milk, especially the very early milk called colostrum, is better for preventing and treating low blood sugar than formula. Most often, if the mother gets good help with breastfeeding, the baby is protected by breastfeeding (at the breast, because skin to skin contact also helps prevent low blood sugar).

Babies with Jaundice

Mothers whose baby has jaundice in the first few days, are often forced to supplement their babies with formula, or even take the baby off the breast altogether because the health professionals "helping her", think that breast milk causes jaundice. **Breastmilk does not cause jaundice**. What causes higher than average levels of bilirubin (the yellow pigment that gives the yellow colour to the baby's skin) in the *majority* of healthy newborn babies of that age is that the baby is *not getting enough breast milk*. And the answer to treating jaundice in the first instance should not be formula in a bottle, but rather helping the mother breastfeed better and get more milk to her baby. Watch a video on www.ibconline.ca of a baby drinking very well at the breast even though he is somewhat jaundiced. Even though he is 10% below birth weight, this is irrelevant because he is drinking so well. Did he do well after leaving hospital? Yes, he did, breastfeeding exclusively.

In the first few days, it is often so easy to turn inadequate breastfeeding around and make it work well and even prevent problems in the first place. But, unfortunately, too many mothers and babies are not getting that help. And the worst of it all is that because the baby's jaundice decreases rapidly once the baby is being formula fed, this "proves" to the health providers that they were right, that the breastmilk caused the jaundice. In fact, the reason the jaundice decreases is that the baby now gets more milk. Could this decrease have been accomplished by helping the mother breastfeed more effectively? Yes, but it happens only rarely that mothers receive this help and the default treatment of jaundice is formula feeding by bottle. It is just so much easier and takes so much less time to tell the mother to feed the baby formula.

True, there are other causes of early onset jaundice than the baby feeding poorly. Hemolysis (an abnormally rapid breakdown of red blood cells), will cause higher than average bilirubin levels, but it is not *breastfeeding* that is causing the elevation of the bilirubin. Of course, poor feeding can combine with hemolysis to cause even higher levels of bilirubin, but part of the treatment should be to help the mother with breastfeeding, not, in the first instance giving the baby formula and blaming breastmilk as the cause of the problem. There are other causes, such as infection in the baby or the baby having a bowel obstruction, but these are unusual causes and again, it's not the breastmilk that causes the problem.

This baby is breastfeeding very well, shown by the very obvious pauses in the chin. But he is 10% below birth weight and the mother is under pressure to supplement, strictly on the basis of the weight. This is so wrong, especially since basing the adequacy of breastfeeding on weight is unreliable, especially if the mother received a large amount of intravenous fluids during labour and birth. And mothers often receive a lot of intravenous fluids during labour and birth.

The Baby with a Cleft Palate

Mothers are told that if their baby has a cleft palate then they cannot breastfeed and should not bother even trying. True, many can't latch on to the breast, *but some can.* But one thing is certain; if one doesn't try, breastfeeding can't happen.

Go to www.ibconline.ca to watch videos showing babies with cleft palate drinking from the breast.

Ten Percent Weight Loss

Mothers are told that if their baby loses more than 10% of his birth weight the baby must have formula by bottle. But the notion of 10% weight loss meaning something is based on nothing scientific and results in many babies being unnecessarily supplemented and, as a result, much too often ending up only bottle feeding. This occurs not only because of the early use of bottles which interferes with the baby's latching on, but also because the mother has been frightened into believing her baby just missed getting severely dehydrated, seriously sick, and even dying. Again, the mother and baby getting good hands on help can change the situation dramatically for the better. People sometimes act as if getting the baby fed and the baby being breastfed were mutually exclusive. The goal of helping mothers should be to get the baby fed by improving breastfeeding. Health professionals need to start looking at the long term effects of their interventions, not just grabbing at the quick fix which formula feeding seemingly offers. More on why percent weight loss is not only meaningless, but damaging to breastfeeding.

Breast Reduction Surgery

Mothers are told that if they have had breast reduction surgery, they won't be able to breastfeed. Maybe most won't be able to breastfeed *exclusively*, but they can still breastfeed with additional properly screened donated breast milk or formula as supplements. And the baby can be at the breast, without receiving bottles, the supplement given with a lactation aid at the breast. Supplementing while the baby is still on the breast is important because, aside from the baby continuing to get more milk from the breast even as the baby is being

30

supplemented, but also, very importantly, breastfeeding is so much more than breastmilk. It is a close, intimate physical and emotional relationship between two people who are usually very much in love with each other. The value of that relationship is not measured by how much breastmilk the mother can produce or the baby receives, and it is important that people start seeing breastfeeding in its various forms. If the baby cannot receive only breastmilk, the baby can, nevertheless, breastfeed exclusively with a lactation aid at the breast. Breastmilk is one thing, breastfeeding is another. Breastfeeding is an act, a relationship. Breastmilk is milk, a very special milk, yes, but breastmilk in a bottle is not breastfeeding.

Mothers Prescribed Medication while Breastfeeding

Too many mothers are told they must interrupt or stop breastfeeding for medications they are taking. With the exception of a very few, usually infrequently used drugs, the mother can and should continue breastfeeding. Furthermore, many of the problematic drugs could be substituted by other equally effective drugs. The vast majority of drugs don't get into the milk in quantities that are harmful to the baby, the amounts being vanishingly small. There are some drugs that don't get into the milk at all and yet mothers are told they will harm their babies if they continue breastfeeding. In any case, the real question is this: Which is safer for the baby, breastfeeding with tiny amounts of drug in the milk (and the amounts are almost always tiny) or formula? Given the risks of *not* breastfeeding, in the vast majority of cases, breastfeeding is safer for the baby.

Access and Custody Cases

Judges dealing with access and custody cases, much too frequently, do not include the needs of the breastfed baby or toddler in their decisions, even though the guiding principle in these cases is, at least in theory, the best interests of the child. Both the father and the mother could be accommodated in terms of spending time with the baby or toddler if the judge realized that breastfed babies and toddlers are *different* from bottle fed babies and toddlers. And breastfed *toddlers* are even more different than the baby. Whether one

31

agrees or not about toddlers breastfeeding, the breastfed toddler derives security and comfort, and yes, love, from breastfeeding, as does the baby, by the way. As mentioned previously breastfeeding is not just about nutrition, a notion that is obviously foreign to so many people, including judges. For the toddler, being forced from the breast can be extremely disturbing emotionally. And it won't be easy for the mother, or the father either for that matter.

Child Protection Services

In many areas, the child protection services are a huge problem for breastfeeding mothers and their babies. Instead of mothers getting help to continue breastfeeding, what the mothers usually get is "Stop breastfeeding, give formula, or we will apprehend your child". These workers just do not understand, they are not trained to understand, they refuse to understand. They do not realize that help, for the mother and baby or toddler, is possible. One recent case I saw was that of a 6 month old baby who definitely was not gaining weight well. I saw the mother and baby and saw that the best way to deal with the situation was to have the mother start food for the baby (after all, the baby was 6 months old) and to increase breastmilk intake by feeding the baby on both breasts at a feeding (she had been told by a lactation consultant to feed on one breast only at each feeding which is a bad idea). The baby started to gain weight well, quite well, but the child protection services were unhappy. The mother didn't listen to the "child protection workers" and the mother was supposed to give formula. So, the baby was taken away from the mother, even though the baby started to gain weight based on our approach. They showed her, didn't they?

The Bottom Line?

These issues are just a few of dozens of situations when mothers are unnecessarily told they must stop breastfeeding; in fact, *must* stop breastfeeding, or else. Most of the time, the problems could have been prevented in the first place or treated without using formula or stopping breastfeeding. But most of the time, the mothers do not get the help they need.

We are not saying that breastfeeding will always work well, even with the best of help, but a lot more mothers and babies could be doing a lot better.

If we went through all the situations we hear about on a daily basis, situations where mothers do not have the right to breastfeed even though they made an informed decision to do so, we would be writing something rather longer than War and Peace. Even if we just went into details regarding the above mentioned problems, it would take a book – however, many situations and answers are described in other chapters of this book, many answers can be found in our information sheets or in our blogs.

WHY ARE BREASTMILK AND FORMULA NOT THE SAME?

Is formula really the same as breastmilk as the formula companies tell us?

There are many people, including many health professionals, who argue that there is no difference between breastmilk and formula now that so many "improvements" in formula have been made and a few previously missing ingredients in formula have been added. However, at the biochemical level, formula is not the same as breastmilk; no formula is even close.

If you take a look at a can of formula and the list of ingredients, it is patently obvious that breastmilk contains many times more "ingredients" than formula, *important* ingredients. Breastmilk contains living cells, stem cells, white cells, immune factors and antibodies which cannot be added to formula. And that's just the beginning. As well, not on the list of ingredients on the formula can are *undesirable* ingredients such as unacceptably high levels of aluminum, arsenic and cadmium (see below).

Most people would readily admit that powdered cow's milk which is re-constituted with hot water is just not the same as fresh milk. But many people have an emotional need to believe that formula is just the same as breastfeeding.

Formula and breastmilk are not at all the same, not even close

Formula company advertising has tried for well over 150 years, starting with Nestlé, to convince parents, and health professionals, that their formulas are the same as breastmilk. The first photo below shows an ad from the late 1890s, which states, in French, "Artificial Milk Feeding", but uses the word in French normally used for "breastfeeding" (*allaitement*). Sneaky, no?

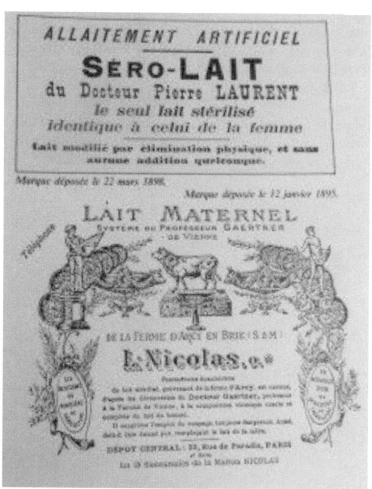

The makers of this formula believed that their formula is exactly the same as mother's milk. Really? Did they really believe it?

And what else does it say? *"le seul lait stérilisé identique à celui de la femme"*: The only sterilized milk **identical** to a woman's milk!!! Incidentally, breastmilk is not sterile and contains many different bacteria. Studies have shown that several hundred different bacteria are *normally* found in breastmilk, though not all in every mother's milk. This is important and *not a bad thing*, and in fact is good for the proper development of the baby's **microbiome** (gut flora) and not something to worry about.

There are many similar ads from that time and so, by the beginning of the 20th century, formula was being widely advertized as just like breastmilk. This misleading advertising has always been essential to formula company sales because otherwise it would have been difficult to convince people to use formula, not only in situations where it might be medically indicated, but also, used massively and unnecessarily as it is used now. Formula being "just like breastmilk" has even become a way for formula companies to compete among different formula brands using words like "closer to breastmilk than ever".

What does the next photo tell us?

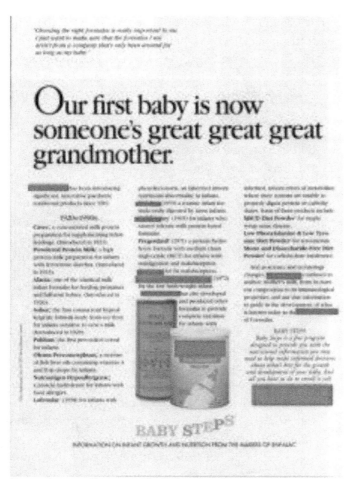

Formulas are "improved" all the time but never equal breastmilk

The ad states that "our formula" has been around since your great great great grandmother's time, presumably in order to make us believe that this company has a lot of experience in making formulas. The ad then goes on to list all the improvements that the manufacturer has made since that time. But note that this ad was printed in the 1990s before:

- *Before* DHA (docosahexaenoic acid), and ARA (arachidonic acid), compounds which have *always* been in breastmilk, were added to formulas, but only after this ad was published. Now that they have been added to formulas **there is no evidence that they have the same effect as when they are in breastmilk** and it has now been shown that they may be harmful in formula. They have been added to some formulas without ever being tested. Because just adding stuff to formula doesn't mean it works in the same way as the ingredient works in breastmilk.

- *Before* the protein content of formulas was reduced because of evidence that too much protein in formulas increases the risk of childhood obesity. However, even now, formulas still contain too much protein, compared to what is in breastmilk and what the baby absorbs from breastmilk. The studies have convinced even the formula manufacturers enough that they have lowered the amount of protein in their formulas. But instead of saying "sorry, we didn't know", they use the lowered concentration of protein to say how wonderful the new formulas are.

- *Before* nucleotides were added to formula (the formula manufacturers made a big deal out of nucleotides in the 1990s, though the importance of nucleotides in formulas has yet to be shown to do much of anything good at all). Nucleotides have always been in breastmilk. We recall a meeting at the Hospital for Sick Children where one of the pediatricians, a specialist in infant nutrition spoke about the importance of nucleotides in the formulas. When asked by one of the pediatricians if nucleotides were really important additions to formulas, he stated that definitely, very important, implying it was a revolutionary change. And why do we not hear about nucleotides in formula now? Basically, because the revolution was a bust.

- *Before* oligosaccharides, the much-vaunted prebiotics, were added to formulas and that formula companies made such a big deal about in the last decade. Oligosaccharides have *always* been in breastmilk.

- *Before* probiotics were added to formulas. Mothers are buying probiotics by the handful to give to their babies. Breastmilk has *always* contained probiotics.

- *Before* most "special formulas" were made for things like spitting up and "allergy".

Think about what this means. It means that formulas that were touted as "just like breastmilk" in the 1890s as well as 1990s were "improved" by all sorts of changes since then. It means that *if* these changes were so important to babies' health, then what about all the babies who received "unimproved formulas" all the way back to your great great great grandmother's time? These formulas were inadequate, likely even harmful.

And what about all those dozens, perhaps even hundreds of other compounds in breastmilk which have not been added and which are unlikely ever to be added? And those compounds yet to be discovered? Breastmilk is a very complex, *living* fluid, the ingredients of which interact with other ingredients in breastmilk to improve the absorption of desirable ingredients, to augment immune function, to decrease inflammation, to help repair damage to cells and much more. And we are just beginning to understand *how* complex, as new ingredients are discovered and how they interact is worked out. For example, everyone seems to know there are antibodies in breastmilk. But there are lots more immune factors in breastmilk than antibodies. And the immune factors interact with each other, work together, to help protect the baby from getting sick.

A mother's milk is unique, made uniquely by a mother for her unique baby

Yes, it is true, every mother makes milk which is different than any other mother. That is because, like all physiological fluids (blood, for example), milk varies from person to person and from one day to another day, and even during the same day. As an example, the amount of sodium in your blood may vary normally quite widely, *normally*, by as much as 15%, depending on how thirsty you are, how much you were sweating in the heat of the day, how much sodium was in your lunch and other factors as well. That's just one example.

We know also that colostrum, the first milk, is very different from the later milk, the milk we seem to consider "real" breastmilk. *Very* different and it even looks different. Yet formula companies and many doctors tell us that formula is a good milk for babies to drink during the first few days. Nobody seems even to question this assumption. And in quantities that far exceed what the baby would get from the breast. More is not necessarily better.

Aside from the much-heralded nucleotides, which play only a very minor role in protecting the baby against infection, formulas contain nothing else that protects babies or toddlers against **infection**. Okay, a few formulas have recently had milk fat globule membrane added to the mix. And milk fat globule membrane are also immune factors, but have effects not only within the immune system, but also on brain structure and function and intestinal development. However, there is no evidence that they actually do what they are supposed to do when ingested from a *formula* milieu, rather than from breastmilk.

Antibodies are only one of many immune factors present in breastmilk that are not present in formulas. Breastmilk contains lactoferrin that is so important to immunity that the formulas are jumping on the lactoferrin bandwagon to discover how to include it in their products. And breastmilk also contains the following immune factors: lysozyme (an enzyme that attacks bacteria and kills them by destroying their cell wall), mucins, lactadherin, bifidus factor and *many* others. And probably many others are yet to be discovered. These immune factors do not just sit there; *they work together*, in beautiful harmony, like the instruments in a symphony orchestra, in reaction to the various bacteria, viruses and funguses to which the mother, and thus also the baby, are exposed. This is *targeted* immunity, very *specific* immunity to what is in the baby's environment, which, of course, includes the mother's environment since mothers and babies are in very close contact much of the time. Even if the immune factors could be added to formulas, they could not "cooperate" as they do in breastmilk. They would not be able to react to infection, because *it's the mother*, through her breastmilk who produces these immune factors *in response to* infection or more accurately, in response to exposure to infectious agents even if she does not become ill with an infection. Breastmilk is a living, dynamic fluid.

Breastmilk contains alpha lactalbumin, which, in the presence of fat in the baby's stomach, is changed to **HAMLET** (human alpha lactalbumin made lethal to tumour cells), which exercises broad anti-tumor activity, (no relation to the Prince of Denmark).

And breastmilk varies from morning to evening, from day to day, from week to week. Because of this, it will never be duplicated by any formulas.

Furthermore, breastmilk is full of anti-inflammatory factors, which decrease inflammation in the baby. Inflammation can cause tissue damage and inflammation occurs as a result of the "battle" of immune factors against bacteria or viruses. As a result of the anti-inflammatory factors and the huge numbers of "good" bacteria in the intestinal tract of the breastfed baby, breastmilk helps prevent the inflammatory reactions which normally would occur when immune factors fight off microbes. In this way, breastmilk decreases the risk of tissue damage of the intestines and is probably one of the reasons breastfed premature babies are less likely to get a serious, potentially life-threatening condition called necrotizing enterocolitis.

There are dozens, if not hundreds of immune factors and other *important* components in breastmilk that are not present in formulas. Just to mention two; one, already mentioned above, an important fairly recently discovered immune factor called milk fat globule membrane. Oh, this is hot stuff and the formula companies have worked feverishly to include milk fat globule membrane into their milk. And some formulas now contain milk fat globule membrane, and the formula advertising now tells us how important this immune factor is, hoping we will forget that all the other formulas before the new ones didn't have milk fat globule membranes. And the other? Stem cells! The mind boggles thinking how stem cells in breastmilk could be used to help in clinical medicine and what they do in the baby's body.

A mother exposed to infection helps protect the baby

See my article in **Scientific American from 1995**. The article explains how breastfeeding protects babies against infection and why it is important to keep babies breastfeeding when the mother has an infection, and when the baby has an infection, including the common infection we get emails about all the time, methicillin resistant *Staphylococcus aureus* (MRSA). Yes, the sick mother protects her baby if she continues breastfeeding. And the sick breastfed baby gets better more quickly by breastfeeding. The following photos from my article show how breastfeeding protects the baby when the mother gets an infection.

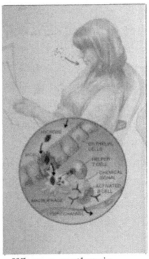

When a mother is exposed to a virus or bacterium, special cells called M cells absorb the bacterium or virus and send information to cells that will travel to the breast and start to add **specific** *antibodies against the bacterium or virus to the breastmilk.*

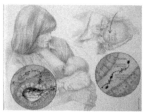

Specific antibodies are secreted into the milk and help to protect the baby against the very infection to which the mother was exposed.

Also hot these days is the **microbiome**, all the bacteria that are part of us, not just in the gastrointestinal tract. Formula fed babies and breastfed babies have very different bacteria in their intestines and elsewhere. And what difference does it make? The microbiome may determine the child's:

- Development including neurological and cognitive development

- Immune function

- Protection against various pathogens

- Digestive function

- Stress levels

- And who knows what else? We are just starting to plumb the secrets about the difference your microbiome makes to health and development

As **one article suggests**:

"We are only beginning to appreciate the potential health benefits that could be accrued from this venture across diagnostic, preventative and treatment realms. We look forward with great anticipation to this transformed appreciation of how our microbial wealth during early life primes for health in adulthood."

With regard to brain development, an interesting article was published in 2013. The authors did magnetic resonance imaging (MRI) in children aged 10 months to 4 years and compared the development of the white matter of the brain in breastfed versus formula fed babies and also looked at how the duration of breastfeeding influences the development of white matter. What do they write? "Breastfed children exhibited increased white matter development in later maturing frontal and association brain regions. Positive relationships between white matter microstructure and breastfeeding duration are also exhibited in several brain regions, that are anatomically consistent with observed improvements in cognitive and behavioral performance measures. While the mechanisms underlying these structural differences remain unclear, our findings provide new insight into the earliest developmental advantages associated with breastfeeding and support the hypothesis that breast milk constituents promote healthy neural growth and white matter development."

Are there things in formula that should not be there?

Of course, here is a quote from an article about **aluminum in formula**. The authors, Shelle-Ann M Burrell and Christopher Exley state: There is (still) too much aluminium in infant formulas *BMC Pediatrics* 2010; 10:63. These authors are not crazed breastfeeding radicals. In their article, they write *"Infant formulas are integral to the nutritional requirements of preterm and term infants"*. Well, we disagree with infant formulas being *integral* to the nutritional requirements of preterm and term infants. Breastfeeding is integral, yes, but not formula. But then they go on to say *"While it has been known for decades that infant formulas are contaminated with significant amounts of aluminium there is little evidence that manufacturers consider this to be a health issue. Aluminium is non-essential and is linked to human disease. There is evidence of both immediate and delayed toxicity in infants, and especially preterm infants, exposed to aluminium and it is our contention that there is still too much aluminium in infant formulas."*

For those who are fond of exotic foods, infant formulas have been found on occasion to contain:

- Beetle parts and beetle larvae

- Pieces of glass

- Metal shavings

- Melamine — due to adulteration of milk by greedy people resulting in many babies in China falling seriously ill

Do humans make mistakes?

Of course they do. And over the years there have been dozens of recalls of formula due to mistakes made in the manufacture of formula. Here are some examples:

Baby formula recalled after 3 infant deaths

An Israeli company partly owned by the American food giant H.J. Heinz has recalled a kosher infant formula after three babies died of nervous disorders and 10 others were hospitalized.

The announcement on Saturday by the company, Remedia, set off a wave of hysteria, and prompted a special religious ruling allowing the notification of ultra-Orthodox Jews on the Sabbath. The recall also affected Orthodox Jewish communities in the United States, where the soy-based formula is sold.

Remedia, whose baby products are found in virtually every Israeli supermarket, said it had slightly altered the makeup of the formula in June to bring it into "accordance with the scientific developments in the field."

Health Ministry officials said the revamped formula lacked Vitamin B1, or thiamine, although the packaging says the vitamin is included.

B vitamins are essential for the development and functioning of the nervous system.   **(AP)**

When mistakes are made, it can be very serious for the baby.

And arsenic in baby formula? **This story**, from October 2017, much more recent than the article of illness in babies in Israel, states that 80% of baby formulas in the US contain measurable amounts of arsenic. And cadmium as well, which is also of concern.

And in December 2017, **salmonella in formula** resulting in a world wide recall of infant formula by the formula manufacturer Lactalis. And, it seems, by mid

2018, everyone seems to have forgotten about it. How do the formula companies get away with it? How is it we forget so quickly?

So? Formula just like breastmilk?

What an incredible statement. Anyone who says such a thing is either completely ignorant of the biochemistry of breastmilk and formula and doesn't know what they are talking about or is plain saying nonsense for political reasons. And if formulas and breastmilk are that different, then they almost certainly have very different effects on the baby and the mother. Just pretending it ain't so don't make it so.

And these differences do not make a difference for the baby or the mother? Some people claim that the studies do not prove there is a difference between breastfed and formula fed babies. Here is the truth: You don't take the normal, the physiological and have to prove that it is better than the artificial. Formula feeding is an intervention, and in medical terms, you have to prove an intervention safe and *of benefit* before it can be recommended.

"But not all women can breastfeed exclusively..."

So yes, what about the women who can't breastfeed exclusively? In fact, most women these days "cannot breastfeed" because they are undermined in their ability to do so. **Hospital routines around labour and birth,** separation of mothers and babies, early introduction of bottles and poor advice from health professionals all together result in so many mothers who "cannot breastfeed" and are disappointed in breastfeeding when they should direct their disappointment at our medical system. If they had had **normal births,** and good help from the beginning, most such mothers would be very successful at breastfeeding.

For the above reasons, breastfeeding has a reputation of being difficult, tiring, **painful,** when, in fact, it should not be difficult, tiring and painful for most mothers. When breastfeeding works as it should, or should have been, it is easy, relaxing and **painless.**

And mothers who cannot breastfeed because of certain **infections** or **other diseases** they might have? Mothers are frequently told they cannot breastfeed for illness and many doctors think they are doing mothers a favour by giving them an excuse to stop breastfeeding. This is medical thinking all too often, that breastfeeding is a burden and mothers will appreciate being told they don't have to carry this burden. Almost never do mothers need to stop for these reasons and had they had good help and encouragement from their doctors, they would not have found breastfeeding a burden.

In truth, my dear doctors, most women *do want to breastfeed* and they are often prevented from breastfeeding by incorrect information on breastfeeding and **illness** or **medications**. Almost never do mothers need to stop for these reasons – HIV, for example, is no longer a reason not to breastfeed nor are many other viral or bacterial infections.

Having surgery is not a reason to stop or even interrupt breastfeeding most of the time. And mothers who cannot breastfeed because of **medications** they are taking? Only rarely do they need to stop because of medications they are taking and frequently it is possible when a drug truly is of concern, to prescribe other similarly effective medications which are compatible with continued breastfeeding. For example, methotrexate is a drug frequently used to treat an ectopic pregnancy (tubal pregnancy). One or two doses will usually result in "cure". And if the mother receives only one or two doses, there is no reason to interrupt breastfeeding. However, methotrexate is also used for long periods of time (months and years) to treat such diseases as rheumatoid arthritis. In this situation it should be considered unsafe for the baby. But another drug, azathioprine can be used long term instead of methotrexate.

Physicians, however, tend to be very conservative. They like to treat illness the way that they always have treated certain illnesses, and too often do not take the needs of the breastfeeding mother and baby into consideration. They should! It should be an integral part of their thinking about treatment of this special group of patients.

But it is true, even if we had perfect labour and birth for every mother, perfect support immediately after the birth and continued support after the immediate postpartum period, some mothers, a small percentage, still would not be able to manage to breastfeed exclusively. And not *all* illnesses will allow mothers to continue breastfeeding and not *all* medications taken by the mother are safe for the baby. And **some illnesses in babies** result in their not being able to be breastfed, usually *rare* inborn errors of metabolism such as galactosemia with very low levels of infant enzyme.

But most such mothers and babies could avoid using formula if we concentrated on developing a widespread system of breastmilk banks so that every mother who needs breastmilk but cannot produce enough would have access to breastmilk. Every hospital should have a breastmilk bank just as they have blood banks. Don't say it's not realistic. If you had asked the same question in 1917 about blood banks, you would have been told it is not realistic to have blood available to everyone who needed blood. This is a question of whether breastmilk instead of formula is seen as a priority and whether we truly understand how different they are.

When talking about women who "cannot" breastfeed, it is often not mentioned how little is done to help them with breastfeeding and to increase their milk supply. If a woman gives her baby supplements, she should be told of all her options – not only formula but banked breastmilk and donor breastmilk so she can make an informed choice. Additionally, when supplementing in a way that does not interfere with breastfeeding, that is, with a **lactation aid at the breast**, the mother is still breastfeeding. It is possible to continue breastfeeding even when supplementing and when the **baby begins to eat food** to achieve a point at which supplementing stops and the baby is breastfed and fed food just like any other breastfeeding baby.

And one more thing, last, but certainly not least. The act of breastfeeding is different from bottle feeding. **Breastfeeding is a close intimate, physical and emotional relationship** between two people in love. And for that, it is not necessary to have a full supply.

HOW BIRTHING PRACTICES MAY AFFECT BREASTFEEDING (PART 1)

Why do so many mothers have difficulty with breastfeeding? A large part of the reasons is that though we tend to believe that breastfeeding should be natural. Most people, particularly most obstetricians, have not yet understood that the "unnatural" way women give birth in much of the world, has an impact on breastfeeding making it difficult and sometimes impossible.

It is important to understand how what is done in the modern health care system to mothers during labour and birth does influence how successful breastfeeding will be. Interventions during labour and birth decrease the chances of breastfeeding starting with ease and without problems. On the other hand, we will admit that many women gave birth with all the interventions possible including a caesarean section and still were able to breastfeed successfully.

Here are just a few of the ways that giving birth in affluent, and not so affluent, societies interfere with breastfeeding.

Epidurals for pain during labour and birth

Intravenous fluids

When a woman is in labour and receiving an epidural, she receives a large amount of fluid by intravenous infusion. The idea is that epidurals may result in a significant drop in the mother's blood pressure and obviously, that is not a good thing. But why do the mothers receive such a large amount of fluid? Three or more litres in 24 hours is not unusual. We have spoken with obstetricians who agree that this very large quantity of intravenous fluid, usually given routinely, is completely unnecessary. Presumably, breastfeeding is not part of the mindset of most anaesthetists or obstetricians.

What is the problem with so much intravenous fluid given to the mother?

When the mother gets such large quantities of fluid, so does the baby, proportionally, and at least a couple of studies have shown that the more fluid the mother receives, the more likely the baby is to lose 10% of his birth weight. And in many hospitals 10% decrease from birth weight automatically means supplementation, usually by bottle, though there has never been any good proof that10% weight loss, rather than 8% or 12% actually means something. But partly because of the intravenous fluids the mother and baby received, evaluating the adequacy of breastfeeding by % weight loss is absurd and leads only to bad practices with regard to breastfeeding. This study by Chantry CJ, Nommsen-Rivers LA, Peerson JM, *et al., Excess weight loss in first-born breastfed newborns relates to maternal intrapartum fluid balance Pediatrics* 2011;127:e171-e179 showed that a greater weight loss in the first few days (more than 10%) was significantly related to the amount of fluids the mother received during labour and birth. This study by Noel-Weiss J *et al., Iatrogenic newborn weight loss: knowledge translation using a study protocol for your maternity setting International Breastfeeding Journal* 2011;6:10 showed the same thing and the authors emphasized the importance of clinical evaluation of breastfeeding rather than depending only on % weight loss to decide if breastfeeding was going well.

But there is more. When a mother has received large amounts of fluids during labour and birth and after the birth as well, she often retains a lot of that fluid for several days. Not only are her hands and feet often swollen, but also her nipples and areolas will be swollen as well, making it difficult for the baby to latch on well (or at all) and thus unable to stimulate the release of milk from the breast. And besides the baby not getting milk well, a poor latch often leads to sore nipples.

Overall, the use of large amounts of intravenous fluids during labour, birth and after the birth often results in early introduction of bottles to babies, early supplementation with formula, and separation of mother and baby (many babies are taken to special care for more than 10% weight loss). Overall, this is the first step for many mothers and babies on the road to breastfeeding failure.

What the mother and baby really need is not automatic bottles and formula which is what is done in too many hospitals, but rather, they need good help with breastfeeding from experienced, skilled nurses and lactation consultants. This includes good help with latching on and the use of breast compression to get more milk to the baby. If the mother has swollen nipples and areolas and it is difficult to achieve a good latch, then reverse pressure softening of the areolas and nipples may help.

What the mother doesn't need, but too often receives, is a nipple shield.

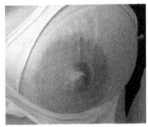

This mother has swelling of the breast, the nipple and areola, due to retention of fluid. This makes it difficult for the baby to latch on. The result? The baby does not get milk well and the mother's nipples are sore. And too often the mother gets started on a nipple shield.

More on % weight loss

Different scales weigh differently. We have seen two scales weigh 400 grams (14 ounces) different for the same baby weighed minutes apart. Most scales are not that far off, but we have seen two scales by the same manufacturer, *the exact same model,* weigh the same baby 85 grams (3 ounces) different and this is probably not unusual. 85 grams for a 3 kg (6lb 10oz) baby is almost 3% so that a baby may lose or gain 3% of his birth weight depending on which scale he was weighed on first. Note that most babies are weighed first in delivery and then, *on another scale*, in postpartum.

Errors in reading the scale or marking down the weight are not rare. We have documented one baby who was weighed at birth at 2.58 kg (5lb 11oz) and 5 hours later weighed 3.1 kg (6lb 13oz). Normally, babies are not weighed every 5 hours, but undoubtedly what happened was that someone looked at the baby when he was at 5 hours old and thought "This baby couldn't possibly weigh only 2.58 kg". But what if the weighs were taken the other way around? Going from 3.1 kg at birth to 2.58 kg the next day is a loss of 17%.

Drugs used during epidural anaesthesia

Anaesthetists generally will tell mothers that the drugs used during epidural anaesthesia do not affect the baby. For those who have seen the difference between babies who were born without epidural or spinal anaesthesia and those born with such anaesthesia, there is no need for proof. The difference between a baby who has not received any drugs from the epidural, who is alert, looking for the breast and ready to crawl to the breast, and a baby drugged by medication, who is sleepy and not interested in the breast is obvious.

But you need studies? Here is a list of studies that shows that babies are indeed affected by the drugs used in epidural anaesthesia.

Brimdyr K, Cadwell K, Widström A-M *et al.* The Association Between Common Labor Drugs and Suckling When Skin-to-Skin During the First Hour After Birth. *Birth* 2015;42(4):319-328

Moisés EC, de Barros Duarte L, de Carvalho Cavalli R, *et al.* Pharmacokinetics and transplacental distribution of fentanyl in epidural anesthesia for normal pregnant women. *Eur J Clin Pharmacol* 2005;61(7):517–522

Ransjö-Arvidson AB, Matthiesen AS, Lilja G, *et al.* Maternal analgesia during labor disturbs newborn behavior: Effects on breastfeeding, temperature, and crying. *Birth* 2001;28(1):5–12

Wiklund I, Norman M, Uvans-Moberg K, *et al.* Epidural analgesia: Breast-feeding success and related factors. *Midwifery* 2009;25(2):e31–e38

Beilin Y, Bodian CA, Weiser J, *et al.* Effect of labor epidural analgesia with and without fentanyl on infant breast-feeding: A prospective, randomized, double-blind study. *Anesthesiology* 2005;103(6):1211–1217

Dozier AM, Howard CR, Brownell EA, *et al.* Labor epidural anesthesia, obstetric factors and breastfeeding cessation. *Matern Child Health J* 2013;17(4):689–698

Torvaldsen S, Roberts CL, Simpson JM, *et al.* Intrapartum epidural analgesia and breastfeeding: A prospective cohort study. *Int Breastfeed J* 2006;1:24

Fever in the mother

When mothers receive epidurals, the longer they have the epidural the more likely they are to get fever.

Lieberman E, Lang JM, Frigoletto F jr *et al.* Epidural analgesia, intrapartum fever and neonatal sepsis evaluation *Pediatrics*1997;99:415-9

"Use of epidural analgesia during labor is strongly associated with the occurrence of maternal intrapartum fever, neonatal sepsis evaluations and neonatal antibiotic treatment."

Segal, S. *Anesth Analg* 2010;111:1467–75

"Women in labor with epidural analgesia experience a larger increase in temperature and more clinical fever than do women who receive other forms of analgesia."

And what is the result of mothers having fever during the labour and birth? Antibiotics for mother and baby and frequently, transfer of the baby to the special care unit. And in some cases, no breastfeeding or breastmilk for the baby because the mother may have an infection.

HOW BIRTHING PRACTICES AFFECT BREASTFEEDING (PART 2)

In part 1 of this chapter, we discussed how the large amounts of intravenous fluids mothers receive during labour and birth and the drugs used in the epidurals, in many cases result in:

- overhydration of the baby,

- difficulty with latching on to the breast,

- unnecessary supplementation of the baby,

- and the mother potentially getting fever.

All of which can negatively affect the initiation and continuation of breastfeeding.

Birth and breastfeeding are often viewed as two separate and independent events and interventions during labour and birth are frequently done without a true medical indication and without taking into consideration the potential side-effects they will have on breastfeeding. What we do during labour and birth to mothers and babies may have significant effects on breastfeeding success and thus should be done only when there is a clear indication that the interventions are necessary. But far too often interventions during labour and birth are done for what can only be described as questionable reasons. Elective caesarean section comes to mind immediately.

We are not saying that interventions during labour and birth must never be done. That is clearly not true; sometimes interventions are necessary.

However, here are a few more, but not all, of the other birthing practices which may interfere with initiation and continuation of breastfeeding:

Oxytocin (Pitocin)

When giving birth in hospital, almost all mothers will receive oxytocin by intravenous infusion to "help the contractions along and make the labour shorter". But oxytocin infusion often makes the contractions more painful and thus increase the "need" for more interventions during the labour and birth. The oxytocin infusion is also continued after the birth to prevent postpartum bleeding. Mothers labouring at home will not usually receive oxytocin during the labour but will receive a single injection of oxytocin after the birth, to prevent bleeding.

We know that having the baby skin to skin immediately after the birth and having the baby drink at the breast at birth releases oxytocin naturally from the mother's pituitary and decreases the risk of postpartum hemorrhage naturally.

Are there concerns about using oxytocin?

This study by Jonas W, *et al.* Effects of Intrapartum Oxytocin Administration and Epidural Analgesia on the Concentration of Plasma Oxytocin and Prolactin, in Response to Suckling During the Second Day Postpartum *Breastfeeding Medicine* 2009;4:70-82, suggests that oxytocin infusion does indeed cause problems. The authors state: "Oxytocin infusion decreased endogenous oxytocin levels dose-dependently", and "Epidural analgesia in combination with oxytocin infusion influenced endogenous oxytocin levels negatively".

This means that it is quite possible that the mother will have difficulty having milk ejection reflexes (letdown reflexes) in the early days after birth and this may result in the baby not getting enough milk. Given the usual hospital approach to breastfeeding, the baby may get formula supplementation that would not have been necessary.

This study Gu V, Feeley N, Gold I, *et al.* Intrapartum Synthetic Oxytocin and Its Effects on Maternal Well-Being at 2 Months Postpartum. *Birth* 2016;43:28-35 concludes that "Women who were exclusively breastfeeding at 2 months postpartum had received significantly less synOT (synthetic oxytocin) compared with their nonexclusively breastfeeding counterparts. Higher synOT dose was associated with greater depressive, anxious, and somatization symptoms. SynOT dose was not associated with perinatal posttraumatic stress."

This result provides evidence that the difficulties that might arise in the first days as suggested by Jonas and others can have longer term effects, into the second month after birth.

Induction of labour

In some hospitals, labour is induced in at least 1/3 of all mothers, often for questionable indications (labour has not started yet at 41 weeks gestation, for example, or "obstetrician is going on vacation"). What's the problem with inducing labour?

Too often, this is the sequence of events: Induction is frequently followed by other interventions, is then followed by failure of the labour to progress resulting often in cæsarean section.

See this study which suggests exactly that sequence of events: Johnson DP, Davis NR, Brown AJ. Risk of cesarean delivery after induction at term in nulliparous women with an unfavorable cervix *Am J Obstet Gynecol* 2003;188:1565-72

"The induction of labor in nulliparous patients especially those with an unfavorable cervix...is associated with a significantly increased risk of caesarean delivery". And, of course, the motto "once a caesarean, always a caesarean" still holds true in the minds of many, if not most, obstetricians.

Caesarean section

Too many mothers end up getting caesarean sections. In some hospitals in North America particularly in the US, 50% of babies are born by caesarean section. In some countries, Brazil, for example, more than 50% of babies are born by caesarean section. This is medical technology gone insane. And what is the problem with caesarean section?

First of all, caesarean section is *not* minor surgery. And there are complications with *any* surgery, such as infection of the incision and the deeper tissues as well as opening up of the incision days after the surgery (dehiscence of the wound). And pain. Pain not only in the days after birth, but often for weeks after the birth and even longer. These complications are often treated with pain medications and antibiotics and mothers are then told that they cannot breastfeed, and it is simply not true that the mother cannot breastfeed while taking medications needed for this or other indications.

Cæsarean section often results in:

- The mother having difficulties moving and finding a comfortable position in which to breastfeed the baby, especially in the first few days.

- Mothers may then be less willing to breastfeed because of pain and discomfort.

- Increased likelihood of mother-baby separation. In some hospitals, babies born by caesarean section are still routinely being sent to the special care unit, even if the caesarean section was done as a "routine" and not for any true indication. Even if the caesarean was done because of concern for the baby, the baby should stay with the mother skin to skin.

- Increased likelihood of the baby being bottle fed formula as a routine, due to separation.

- The mother is more likely to get medication sometimes without knowing. For example, most mothers are not aware that they receive a shot of antibiotics during the surgery. Or she may receive more antibiotics after the birth, or more oxytocin.

<u>Pain for more than a few days?</u>

This is what this study shows: Declercq E, Cunningham DK, Johnson C, Sakala C. Mothers' reports of postpartum pain associated with vaginal and cesarean deliveries: results of a national survey *Birth* 2008;35(1):16-24

Results: "The most frequently cited postpartum difficulty was among mothers with a cesarean section, 79 percent of whom reported experiencing pain at the incision in the first 2 months after birth, with 33 percent describing it as a major problem and 18 percent reporting persistence of the pain into the sixth month postpartum. Mothers with planned cesareans without labor were as likely as those with cesareans with labor to report problems with postpartum pain."

This should not be surprising. Anyone who has had surgery knows very well that pain may continue for months and even years after the surgery. Pain may not necessarily be present all the time, but pain and come and go, which does not necessarily make it minor.

WHAT IS A GOOD LATCH?

How a baby latches on is very important to the amount of breastmilk the baby receives from the breast. And is also very important to prevent and treat sore nipples and sore breasts in the mother.

There has been a shift in breastfeeding thinking that should have occurred a long time ago. A shift to the "asymmetric". An asymmetric latch. When the mother is able to achieve an asymmetric latch, the baby receives more milk from the breast and the mother is less likely have sore nipples, while at the same time the asymmetric latch *treats* sore nipples. Showing mothers what an asymmetric latch looks like and how to actually latch the baby on with an asymmetric latch, are amongst the first things we do at our clinic when helping mothers with breastfeeding. Together with breast compression, it is a foundation for everything else we do.

Why does the latch make a difference? I think that almost all of us who help mothers prevent and overcome breastfeeding problems will agree that the deeper (or "better") the baby's latch on the breast, the better for mother and baby. It is better from the point of view of mother's having pain or not, and how well the baby gets breastmilk from the breast.

Pain during breastfeeding is a sign the mother needs help; so, if breastfeeding hurts, almost always, the baby's latch is not as good as it could be. Even Candida ("thrush", "yeast") infections, overly diagnosed incidentally, are due to an underlying problem, since *Candida does not grow on normal skin*; the damage to the nipple and areola from a less than adequate latch is usually the underlying problem which is too often ignored and needs to be attended to if we are to provide a permanent solution to Candida or *nipple pain of any kind.* As well, the better the latch, the more breastmilk the baby will get from the breast.

The experience of my time in west Africa provided me with an interesting insight: one of the things I noticed back many years ago was that the mothers were often latching the baby on with what most breastfeeding specialists would consider a poor latch. I discussed this with the person in charge of teaching for the Baby Friendly Hospital Initiative. I wondered why, if how the baby latched on was so important, what explained that mothers we were seeing had babies with really poor latches sometimes and yet neither the mother nor the baby had problems with breastfeeding. True, sore nipples, even there, were considered "normal" but most mothers seemed to overcome their sore nipples. I didn't anticipate her answer: "Yes, quite right, but the mothers in this area are reputed to have their milk drying up very early, usually within the first 4 months".

And we see this problem of late onset decreased milk supply in Toronto as well. And emails I receive from everywhere in the world suggest that the problems mothers are running into are also due to late onset decreased milk supply. Mothers who started off with an abundant milk supply, starting around 3 or 4 months after birth have babies who start acting as if they are not getting fast enough flow of milk from the breast. They pull at the breast, they fuss at the breast and fuss between feedings. They are sucking their fingers much of the time, and they may even refuse to take the breast, especially during the day, though they may feed well and frequently during the night. And all this may occur despite the baby breastfeeding exclusively and even gaining weight well. Which makes it difficult for the mothers to believe their milk supply has decreased – this decrease *being relative* to the copious milk supply the mother had in the beginning. Because this problem is typically the problem of the mother who began with an abundant milk supply.

Because of continued good weight gain in many, the babies are diagnosed with "reflux", or allergy to something in the mother's milk. But these diagnoses can only be made if one does not look at the whole picture and watching to see if the baby is drinking well from the breast or not. Watching the baby at the breast will verify that the baby is pulling, crying, popping off and on the breast when the flow of milk slows.

Go to www.ibconline.ca to watch videos showing babies drinking from the breast or not.

We commonly hear from mothers that they were told the baby's latch was good. However, when we see the mothers and babies at the clinic, it is clear the baby's latch could be much better and we show them how to make a shift to the asymmetric latch.

With the asymmetric latch, the baby's chin is in the breast, but the nose is not. The baby covers more of the areola with his lower lip than his upper lip. The second photo below shows the opposite of the asymmetric latch. And why is one asymmetric latch better than the other?

In the first photo below, the baby has an asymmetric latch, the chin is in the breast, the nose is not. In second photo below, the baby does the opposite – the nose touches the breast and the chin does not. In the first photo, the baby has more of the breast where his lower jaw and gums, and the tongue are.

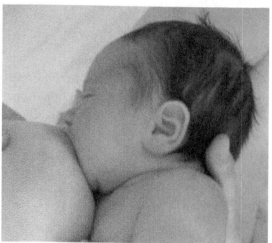

This baby has an asymmetric latch – the chin is in the breast, but the nose does not touch the breast

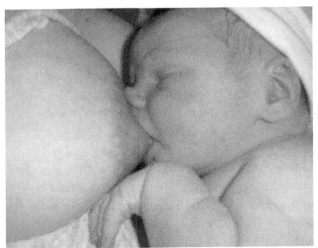

This baby has a poor latch – the opposite of an asymmetric latch. The nose is in the breast, the chin is not.

In second photo, the baby has more of the breast where his maxilla (upper jaw) is. In the first photo, the baby's lower jaw and tongue can stimulate the breast to release its milk, to stimulate rapid flow. In the second photo, the upper jaw *does not move,* so the stimulation of the breast is just not effective since the *lower* jaw and tongue are very shallowly attached to the breast. Furthermore, the baby's tongue is stimulating the nipple, not the breast tissue. The situation becomes even worse if the baby has a tongue tie and thus, the baby's tongue cannot stimulate the breast well.

CAN YOU TELL WHETHER A BABY'S LATCH IS GOOD?

Getting the **best latch possible** when a baby is breastfeeding is crucial for helping mothers with breastfeeding problems and it is one of the skills that we teach mothers at **our breastfeeding clinic**. A good latch is the basis for:

- Helping a mother with sore nipples.

- Helping the baby get more breastmilk from the breast.

- Preventing future problems such as **blocked ducts, mastitis**, late onset decreased milk supply and flow of breastmilk to the baby, late onset sore nipples, "reflux", "allergy to something in the mother's milk".

At our breastfeeding clinic we teach **latching on differently from most others.** We teach the mothers to use an **asymmetric latch**.

What does an asymmetric latch look like? The baby covers more of the areola with his lower lip than his upper lip and the chin is in the breast but the nose doesn't touch the breast. The reason for the baby's nose not touching the breast is not to help the baby breathe better but rather so that the baby's latch is the very best possible and so that the baby will be able to better stimulate the breast with the lower gums and tongue and thus to get as much breastmilk as possible and to prevent or treat the underlying cause of sore nipples.

Take a look at the two photos below labeled photo 1 and photo 2, both are photos of the same baby. Which of the photos shows a better latch – in other words, which of the photos shows a more asymmetric latch?

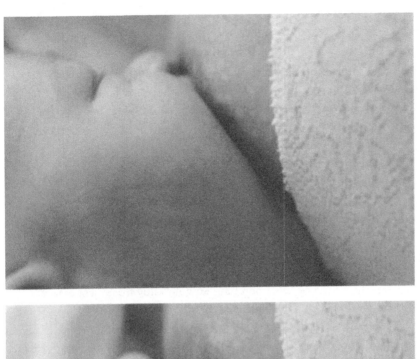

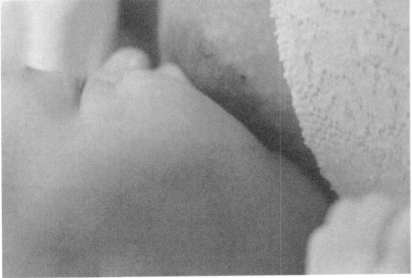

Compare these two photos of the same breastfeeding baby to determine which is an asymmetric latch

You can find the answer if you read on. If you need help with the answer, read the previous chapter with photos which explains **what an asymmetric latch is**.

At our clinic we have more than 33 years experience helping mothers with the asymmetric latch, and our lactation consultants have had training and have developed their skills to use the asymmetric latch to help mothers with a large variety of breastfeeding problems.

ANSWER: When you look at the two photos, photo 1 shows the baby latched on in a "traditional", *symmetric* latch, which often works well, the baby receiving milk well, and the mother is not experiencing problems with breastfeeding, especially sore nipples. In photo 1, the nose is close to the breast and the attachment is "bull's eye" rather than asymmetric. Photo 2 shows an asymmetric latch which is better especially if the mother and baby are having difficulties with breastfeeding. The asymmetric latch works well to prevent problems in the first place. In photo 2, there is a space between the baby's nose and the breast, the baby's head is more tilted back (more extended, to use the medical term) and the baby covers more of the areola with his lower lip than his upper lip with the nipple pointing more towards the roof of the baby's mouth.

The asymmetric latch works better because the baby has more of the breast over his lower gums, and it is the lower part of the mouth that moves and **stimulates the breast to release its milk**. Imagine in photo 2, above, the baby's jaw is moving. In effect, the baby's jaw and tongue are stimulating the breast as if the baby had a much "deeper" latch. Perhaps the next photo illustrates this better.

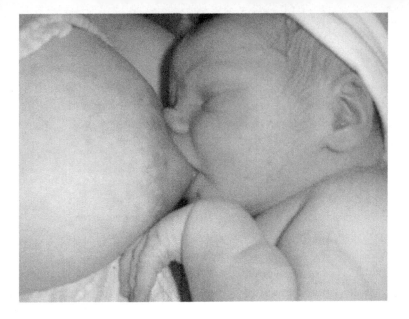

The answer to the question in the beginning of the article is photo 2.

DOES TONGUE TIE CAUSE BREASTFEEDING PROBLEMS?

I don't think there is any doubt that tongue ties can cause breastfeeding problems. And the reason is that the key to successful breastfeeding is for the mother to help the baby achieve **as good a latch as possible**! A good latch results in **pain-free breastfeeding** and the baby getting good flow of milk from the breast. Our experience over many years confirms the importance of tongue tie in causing mothers and babies difficulties with breastfeeding. This, despite many pediatricians who probably have never learned anything about breastfeeding saying that tongue tie does not affect breastfeeding. These same pediatricians often have only one approach to helping mothers with breastfeeding: "give formula". When it comes to breastfeeding, many pediatricians seem to take the stance "I know what I know, and please don't confuse me with facts".

A baby with a tongue tie, cannot have a good latch and cannot exercise the full range of tongue motions necessary to **stimulate the breast to release breastmilk**. There is now sufficient data from several studies that a tongue tie does cause breastfeeding problems. See the studies at the end of this chapter.

Questions that arise:

What is a tongue tie?

A tongue tie exists when the thin piece of tissue, called the frenulum, which connects the tongue to the floor of the mouth, is too thick or too tight so that the mobility of the tongue is restricted. It *may* affect several areas of a person's life but has the greatest implications for breastfeeding because this is when the greatest tongue mobility is necessary for the baby to stimulate the breast properly and receive enough milk from the breast and for the mother to be comfortable breastfeeding and not in pain. It is worthwhile considering that breastfeeding problems are *cumulative*. If the baby has only a tongue tie, it is possible that neither the mother will have nipple pain, nor the baby have difficulty getting enough from the breast. But add to the tongue tie mother's swollen nipples and areolas from overhydration with **intravenous fluids,** separation of mothers and babies, babies getting supplement by bottle etc... And now there is a problem, of which the tongue tie is only one element.

Are there more babies with tongue ties than 50 years ago?

It seems unlikely. Why would that be? The supplementation of the pregnant woman with folic acid to prevent spina bifida has been postulated as a possible cause, but there is no good evidence at all to suggest this as a cause of tongue tie.

People these days get the impression that a huge number of babies are being diagnosed with a tongue tie and wonder why tongue ties were not a problem in the past.

In general, in medicine, we are now able to diagnose more conditions than we were in the past and link them the symptoms people are experiencing. This is the case with tongue tie as well. However, tongue tie is not new, and it has been known for centuries that tongue ties were a problem for breastfeeding and were being corrected in primitive ways by midwives.

Additionally, many more women are breastfeeding now than say, 50 years ago, and so this issue comes to the forefront whereas before it would have been "treated" by giving the baby a bottle of formula, (and still is being "corrected" in this way, unfortunately).

We would like to repeat that problems with breastfeeding are *cumulative* and these days tongue ties are diagnosed in a situation when more babies and mothers are having breastfeeding problems arising from the *almost* universal **interventions during labour and birth** as well as interventions soon after birth, such as giving bottles of formula for **low blood sugar** and **jaundice.** *Most* mothers are not getting **adequate help in the hospital** to **prevent or treat problems** early after birth. And they are looking for **solutions** to their problems and they are **not getting good solutions** from their doctors or most other health professionals. Usually the only solution on offer is "supplement", but many mothers don't accept that "solution" any longer. They rightly want breastfeeding solutions to assure that breastfeeding will continue.

We have only just started, in the past 20 to 25 years, to fully recognize tongue tie as a factor in causing breastfeeding problems. And "we" unfortunately, does not include many physicians and pediatricians. To the point where in some hospitals, nurses and lactation consultants have been forbidden, on pain of dismissal, even to mention the possibility that the baby has a tongue tie to the parents.

Furthermore, now many more mothers don't accept the word of doctors or midwives or lactation consultants that there is no tongue tie or that it is mild and of minimal importance. In fact, our experience is that if the tongue tie is said to be "mild" it is far more than mild and the mothers' problems are far greater than minimal.

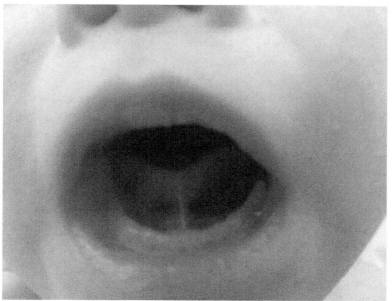

In this case, the doctor did diagnose a tongue tie. (It is so obvious that it could be diagnosed by a 5 year old and it is indeed very tight.), but the doctor said that the tongue tie had nothing to do with the mother's severe nipple pain, but rather was a "cosmetic problem only". What on earth could that mean? The baby has an

ugly tongue?

Many health professionals also were embarrassed years ago about releasing tongue ties for "preventing speech problems". And release of tongue tie to prevent speech problems died out when studies were published that moderate tongue ties do not cause speech problems in languages such as English whose phonemes (sounds) do not require a wide range of tongue mobility. This left many health professionals with a feeling of having been recommending a procedure that had no value. Something like the feeling they had when it was found that the virtually universal tonsillectomy and adenoidectomy in young children was being done too often without a good reason.

In fact, mild tongue tie does not seem to cause problems for native speakers of English or that the "lisp" and speech impediments are minor and thus go unnoticed because of a wide variety of pronunciations of different phonemes (sounds) being tolerated by English speakers. But it does for speakers of many languages where the "r" is "rolled", as in Spanish and many other languages, including Slavic languages and Arabic or where there are other phonemes which require a greater tongue mobility and where tolerance for "wrong pronunciation" is low and a source of ridicule.

An anecdote: When we tell parents that the baby has a tongue tie and they have never heard of this before, we spend a long time explaining to the parents why the tongue tie might be a problem, what is involved in releasing it and what to do about after care (in fact we no longer recommend stretching exercises but are starting to rethink this question also). One day, we saw a family originally from Serbia. The mother had very sore nipples. After I (Dr Jack Newman) examined the baby, I said to the parents that the baby had a tongue tie. The father, instead of asking for a long explanation about this, immediately said "Cut it". I was taken aback, to say the least, as the father asked for no explanation at all. When I asked him why he agreed without explanation, he said that *he* himself had had a tongue tie when he was a child and could not roll his "r" and was mocked in school. At the age of 25 years, he finally had his tongue tie released and he could immediately roll his "r". He did not want his baby to have the same problems as he did.

Do health professionals know how to diagnose tongue tie?

In fact, many, if not most, doctors, nurses, lactation consultants don't know how to diagnose a tongue tie. Diagnosing a tongue tie is about much more than a quick look into the baby's mouth. It is important to feel, for the "feeling" of tightness by sweeping one's finger underneath the baby's tongue from side to side and then trying to lift the tongue to test for upward mobility of the tongue (photo below).

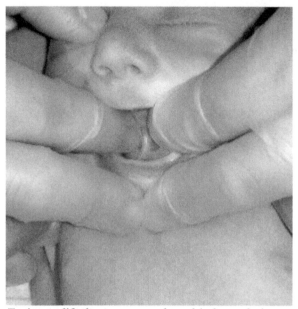

Trying to lift the tongue makes this less obvious tongue tie more obvious. Restriction of upper mobility of the tongue suggests a significant tongue tie. Note, the lactation consultant's right thumb is not resting on the baby's eye.

In the photo below, we see a baby with a tongue tie who does not have an obvious frenulum, never mind a tight one. But the heart shape of the baby's tongue suggests very strongly that the baby has a restriction of upward movement of the tongue.

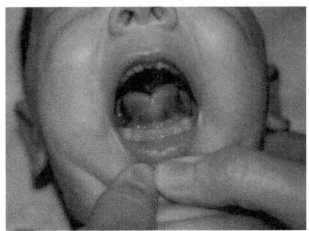

Tongue tie without obvious frenulum. By looking, one does not see a frenulum, so many health providers would say "no tongue tie". We released this baby's tongue tie and the mother's pain resolved.

The diagnosis of a tongue tie in the context of breastfeeding involves a combination of two elements: examination of the baby's tongue and by observing the baby breastfeed in the context of the breastfeeding difficulties the mother and baby are encountering.

Some problems that are caused by or *aggravated* by a tongue tie may include:

1. A baby who is **not latching on**

2. A mother who has **sore nipples** (early on or late onset due to **late onset decreased milk supply,** see below)

3. A baby who is **not getting enough breastmilk from the breast**

4. A baby and mother who are experiencing **late onset decrease in milk supply**

But can't mothers succeed at breastfeeding when their babies have tongue ties?

Of course, and many probably always did succeed in spite of a tongue tie. We have seen mothers and babies at our clinic occasionally where the baby has a very tight tongue tie and yet the mother has no pain and the baby is latching on and getting plenty of milk. If the mother has an abundant supply, there may not be any problems.

However, on the other hand, we see *many* mothers whose 3 or 4 month old babies are reacting to **late onset decreased milk supply** (pulling at the breast, mother with late onset sore nipples, baby even not gaining well any longer, sucking his fingers much of the time, even refusing the breast). We do worry that because of the tongue tie, the mother's milk supply will decrease with time and we are not always sure what to do about the tongue tie.

It should be noted that many mothers believe or are told that they have "oversupply" or an "overactive letdown reflex", but if the baby cannot handle the flow, it's not usually because the flow is too rapid, it's usually because **the baby's latch could be better**. Too often, however, "oversupply" or "overactive letdown reflex" are "treated" with the suggestion that the mother feed the baby on **one breast at each feeding**, or worse, "block feeding" (the baby fed on one breast for several feedings in a row, then fed on the other side, for several feedings in a row). The result? **Late onset decreased milk supply**.

Breastfeeding problems are cumulative, so that, for example, a mother who gets off to a good start with breastfeeding may have no problems in spite of the baby having a tongue tie.

But add to a baby's tongue tie, a mother whose nipples and areolas are swollen from **intravenous fluids given during labour** so the baby latches on poorly or not at all, and so is given bottles and even separated from the mother etc... and now there is a significant problem.

Unrecognized tongue ties, however, are likely reasons for the baby failing to gain weight, for premature weaning and for early introduction of bottles of formula. In the past, people may have seen the symptoms of tongue tie as "the baby didn't want to breastfeed" or "breastfeeding was too painful to bear" or "I just couldn't breastfeed" or "the baby didn't gain weight" or "my milk was not good enough" but may not have recognized the tongue tie as part of the cause.

Our way of releasing tongue ties

We release the tongue ties with scissors, not laser. We see many babies in our clinic whose tongue ties had been previously released with laser and there has been significant re-attachment. Of course, it is possible that re-attachment is less common with laser release, but then we don't usually see those babies who have had laser release, since, presumably, things are going better. But laser release never re-attached? Definitely not true. And laser release takes much longer and hurts the whole time. With scissors, the tongue tie release takes less than a second.

We do not use any anaesthetic. The best anaesthetic is breastfeeding (before the procedure and right after), and we like the mother to stay in the room with us when we release the tongue tie, or just outside by the door if she is squeamish. In this way, the baby can go straight to the breast and usually stops crying immediately. If the baby's tongue and mouth have been anaesthetized, the baby cannot latch on properly or suck well and get relief and comfort from breastfeeding. The baby calming down by breastfeeding usually stops any bleeding as well. And finally, the taste of the anaesthetic by itself is probably unpleasant for the baby.

We do not recommend exercises to prevent re-attachment. We have seen no good evidence that they make a difference. In our experience, also, we have not seen a difference in re-attachment. For a while we were asking some parents to do the exercises and some not to. Though this was not a formal study, we saw an equal incidence of re-attachment with both groups. But there *was* a difference between the two groups, and that was that the re-attachment *tended* to be thicker and less mobile with exercises than without. When exercises were *not* done, the frenulum was thinner and more mobile. Furthermore, the baby and the parents hate the exercises. The exercises are painful for the baby and the parents. Nevertheless, as we constantly do about everything we do in the clinic, we are re-evaluating our position on stretching exercises.

Those who do laser release often recommend 4 to 6 weeks of exercises, several times a day. I just cannot imagine the parents doing that. Even a week later, when we see the baby and mother in followup, when we check the inside of the baby's mouth, very gently, the baby cries.

Releasing a tongue tie

As you will see, it is important have good lighting and to hold the baby well to prevent movement of the baby's head, while at the same time exposing the tongue tie.

Go to www.ibconline.ca to watch videos showing a tongue tie release.

I use scissors to make a snip at 90 degrees to the edge of the frenulum and cut **no more than 1 or 2 mm** and then use the index finger of my left hand to push on the cut so that it tears, in the same way as one cuts cloth. When the tongue tie has been fully released, one sees only a diamond-shaped wound where the frenulum once was.

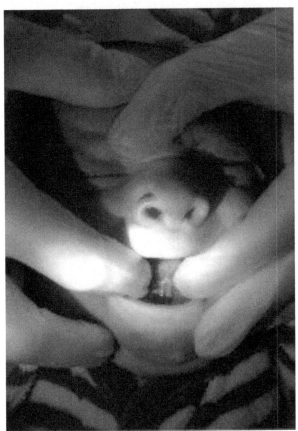

The appearance under the tongue after tongue tie release.

Bleeding is minimal if done this way and almost always stops as soon as the baby goes to the breast.

Helping mothers and babies with breastfeeding problems is about much more than releasing a tongue tie. Mothers need help achieving the **ideal latching on of the baby,** help in the use of other ways of improving the breastfeeding such as **breast compression** and of course, close follow-up. Any health professional who does tongue tie releases but does not have the skills to help the mother and babies with the actual breastfeeding should make sure that the mother does have good help and support and followup.

What are our results? (We follow all mothers and babies about 1 week after the initial release).

1. When a mother has sore nipples, some mothers get immediate and long-lasting pain relief.

2. Some mothers get temporary relief for a few days and then the nipple soreness returns. This is very suggestive that the tongue tie has re-attached.

3. Some babies have re-attachment when we see them on follow-up. However, the mother's pain is still gone or much improved. It seems as if the mother and baby just needed a few days to get "over the hump" and then all is well in spite of the re-attachment. In such a case we would not re-release the tongue tie but ask the mother to watch for signs of **late onset decreased milk supply**.

4. Increased intake of milk by the baby is sometimes very obvious, particularly when the baby's tongue tie is released when he is only a few days old. Once the baby is older than a couple of weeks, the improvement in drinking is more difficult to document easily or immediately because milk supply may decrease rapidly when a baby does not latch on well. Nevertheless, we think that it does help to improve milk intake by the baby over time.

5. When the mother has **late onset decreased milk supply** we prefer to increase the mother's milk supply with **domperidone first**, and then release the tongue tie a week or so later. The problem is that sometimes babies of 3 or 4 months of age will occasionally refuse the breast if the tongue tie is released before the milk supply is increased.

Your doctor/your lactation consultant/you want studies and articles?

Here are several:

1. Geddes DT, Kent JC, McClellan HL, *et al.* **Sucking characteristics of successfully breastfeeding infants with ankyloglossia: a case series.** *Acta Paediatr* 2010;99:301-3

"…these results suggest that some mothers may have particular breast/nipple or milk ejection characteristics that contribute to successful breastfeeding of infants with ankyloglossia."

2.Kumar M, Kalke E. **Tongue-tie, breastfeeding difficulties and the role of Frenotomy.** *Acta Pædiatrica* 2012;101:687-689

"Neonates with tongue-tie are at increased risk for breastfeeding difficulties. An early recognition of this association by primary care provider and prompt referral to a lactation consultant is important. In cases with clearly documented breastfeeding difficulties, frenotomy often results in rapid improvement in symptoms."

3. Hall, DMB, Renfrew MJ. **Tongue tie: Common problem or old wives' tale?** *Arch Dis Child* 2005;90;1211-1215

No abstract, a commentary.

4. Messner AH, Lalakea L, Aby J, Macmahon J, Bair E. **Ankyloglossia. Incidence and associated feeding difficulties.** *Arch Otolaryngol Head Neck Surg.* 2000;126:36-39

"Ankyloglossia, which is a relatively common finding in the newborn population, adversely affects breastfeeding in selected infants."

5. Srinivasan A, Dobrich C, Mitnick H, Feldman P. **Ankyloglossia in Breastfeeding Infants: The Effect of Frenotomy on Maternal Nipple Pain and Latch.** *Breastfeeding Medicine.* 2006;1(4)216-224

"Timely frenotomy and breastfeeding counseling is an effective intervention, improving latch and decreasing nipple pain."

6. Edmunds J, Miles S, Fullbrook P. **Tongue tie and breastfeeding: A review of the literature.** *Breastfeeding Review* 2011;19(1):19-26

"In Australia, initial exclusive breastfeeding rates are 80%, reducing to 14% at 6 months. One factor that contributes to early breastfeeding cessation is infant tongue-tie, a congenital abnormality occurring in 2.8-10.7% of infants in which a thickened, tightened or shortened frenulum is present. Tongue-tie is linked to breastfeeding difficulties, speech and dental problems. It may prevent the baby from taking enough breast tissue into its mouth to form a teat and the mother may experience painful, bleeding nipples and frequent feeding with poor infant weight gain; these problems may contribute to early breastfeeding cessation. This review of research literature analyses the evidence regarding tongue-tie to determine if appropriate intervention can reduce its impact on breastfeeding cessation concluding that, for most infants, frenotomy offers the best chance of improved and continued breastfeeding. Furthermore, studies have demonstrated that the procedure does not lead to complications for the infant or mother."

7. Dollberg S, Botzerb E, Grunis E, Mimouni FB. **Immediate nipple pain relief after frenotomy in breast-fed infants with ankyloglossia: a randomized, prospective study.** _Journal of Pediatric Surgery_ 2006;41,1598-1600

"Frenotomy appears to alleviate nipple pain immediately after frenotomy. We speculate that ankyloglossia plays a significant role in early breast-feeding difficulties, and that frenotomy is an effective therapy for these difficulties."

8. Amir LH, James JP, Beatty J. **Review of tongue-tie release at a tertiary maternity hospital.** _J Paediatr Child Health._ 2005;41:243-245

"Frenotomy is a safe and easy procedure. Infants with a significant tongue-tie that is interfering with breastfeeding have shown an improvement with breastfeeding following frenotomy."

9. Hogan M, Westcott C, Griffiths M. **Randomized, controlled trial of division of tongue-tie in infants with feeding problems.** _J Paediatr Child Health_ 2005;41:246-250

"This randomized, controlled trial has clearly shown that tongue-ties can affect feeding and that division is safe, successful and improved feeding for mother and baby significantly better than intensive skilled support of a lactation consultant."

10. Ballard JL, Auer CE, Khoury JC. **Ankyloglossia: Assessment, Incidence, and Effect of Frenuloplasty on the Breastfeeding Dyad.** *Pediatrics* 2002;110(5).

"Ankyloglossia is a relatively common finding in the newborn population and represents a significant proportion of breastfeeding problems. Poor infant latch and maternal nipple pain are frequently associated with this finding. Careful assessment of the lingual function, followed by frenuloplasty when indicated, seems to be a successful approach to the facilitation of breastfeeding in the presence of significant ankyloglossia."

11. Geddes DT, Langton DB, Gollow I, Jacobs LA, Hartmann PE, Simmer K. **Frenulotomy for Breastfeeding Infants With Ankyloglossia: Effect on Milk Removal and Sucking Mechanism as Imaged by Ultrasound.** *Pediatrics* 2008;122;e188-e194

"Infants with ankyloglossia experiencing persistent breastfeeding difficulties showed less compression of the nipple by the tongue postfrenulotomy, which was associated with improved breastfeeding defined as better attachment, increased milk transfer, and less maternal pain. In the assessment of breastfeeding difficulties, ankyloglossia should be considered as a potential cause."

12. Buryk M, Bloom D, Shope T. **Efficacy of Neonatal Release of Ankyloglossia: A Randomized Trial.** *Pediatrics* 2011;128;280

"We demonstrated immediate improvement in nipple pain and breastfeeding scores, despite a placebo effect on nipple pain. This should provide convincing evidence for those seeking a frenotomy for infants with significant ankyloglossia."

13. Garbin CP, Sakalidis VS, Chadwick LM, *et al.* **Evidence of Improved Milk Intake After Frenotomy: A Case Report.** *Pediatrics* 2013;132:e1413-e1417

"This case study confirms that ankyloglossia may reduce maternal milk supply and that frenotomy can improve milk removal by the infant. Milk-production measurements (24-hour) provided the evidence to confirm these findings." (My comment: I think the authors are incorrect in adding this in the conclusions "This outcome confirms that ankyloglossia was the reason for poor milk transfer from the breast compared with the bottle rather than "nipple confusion.")

BREAST COMPRESSION

We use a number of ways to help mothers and babies breastfeed better when they come to our clinic. One group of babies we see frequently are babies who cry or fuss, are not satisfied after breastfeeding, who need to start drinking more milk or who are already being supplemented.

Amongst the ways we try to help is to show the mother how to **adjust the baby's latch** so that the baby is able to stimulate the release of milk and increase the milk flow to the baby. Another is to show mothers how to use, what we call, breast compressions.

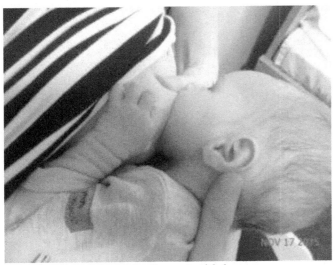

A mother compresses her breast with her left hand to increase milk flow to the baby

I learned about breast compressions when I was working in Africa. I watched mothers compress or squeeze their breasts. They did this almost automatically, but I never really understood why or probably did not even think about what they were doing.

Then, several years ago, when the clinic was still in its early days, a woman from Chile came for advice. She was doing breast compressions as I watched

84

her breastfeed. And so, I asked her why she was doing this. She answered, "Because my mother said I should". I responded that this was a good thing, but why? And she looked at me as if she was wondering why she came to me for help and said, "Because the baby gets more milk…". I truly felt that she left unsaid, "…stupid!" And truly the penny did drop for me and I thought back and finally realized what all those African mothers were doing. And we have used it successfully at the clinic ever since. It is not the only method that we use to increase the intake of milk by the baby, but it is a simple one and one that is very easy to use.

Compression of the breast is an easy and effective method of getting more breastmilk to the baby when the baby is latched on to the breast. A baby is not getting milk from the simply because the baby is latched on and making sucking motions. **Watch a video** on www.ibconline.ca of a **mother of a two day** old baby doing breast compressions.

Go to www.ibconline.ca to watch videos showing mothers doing compressions.

WHEN IT HURTS TO BREASTFEED PART 1

Sore nipples are the problem we see most commonly **at our clinic**, neck and neck with the "baby not getting enough from the breast", though, of course, unfortunately, the two problems often co-exist. At the same time, the baby receiving less milk increases the mother's nipple pain because slow flow of milk from the breast often results in the baby's latch not being as good as it could be. Furthermore, many babies tend to pull away from the breast when the flow of milk is slow, not always letting go, thus adding to the mother's pain.

Sore nipples can almost always be prevented or if they do occur, they can be much more easily treated when the baby is a few days old than when the baby is a few weeks old or even older.

Unfortunately, too many health providers seem to believe that it is normal for breastfeeding to hurt. We strongly disagree with this. Pain tells us something is wrong. But as a result of this belief that breastfeeding "normally" hurts, mothers are told, in various ways, "Just bear with it, it will get better". Okay, sometimes sore nipples do get better spontaneously over the first few weeks, but why should mothers suffer for weeks, when effective treatment is available? As one of our patients was told by a postpartum nurse "You wanted to breastfeed? So just suck it up." On the other hand, one lactation consultant who mentioned to a nurse that she had no pain with her own two day old baby, received the retort "You're just lucky."

The notion that breastfeeding is supposed to hurt, that it is normal for breastfeeding to hurt, is an excuse for not doing anything to help a mother in pain. But something needs to be done. Sore nipples can be agonizingly painful. Unfortunately, too many health providers don't know what to do, don't know how to help and too often blithely state or think: "It can't be that bad if you are continuing to breastfeed."

The latch, the latch, the latch!

86

We don't accept that pain is a normal part of breastfeeding; painful breastfeeding seems to be unique to humans in the mammalian world. There seems to be an idea that, well, if labour hurts, then it's natural that breastfeeding hurts. This is fuzzy thinking. The end of the pain of labour, accompanied by the birth of the baby, is a double joy. Painful breastfeeding is in no way joyful and serves no purpose. Furthermore, **we can help mothers have pain free breastfeeding**

But if breastfeeding hurts, what is the cause? Almost always, the problem is **the way the baby latches on.** And just as a latch can be a cause of the baby **not getting as much milk from the breast as he could,** so can the way a baby latches on can cause the mother sore nipples. Yes, admittedly, even with a terrible latch, a mother may not have sore nipples and if she has an abundant milk supply, things can be **fine, for a while.** But if the mother has sore nipples, the latch definitely is not as good as it could be.

And why is the latch not as good as it could be?

Because of:

1. **How the baby is positioned and latched on.** Babies often have difficulty latching on well in the first days after birth because of the **swelling of the mother's nipples and areolas from the intravenous fluids the mother receives during labour, birth and after.**

2. Using artificial nipples such as bottles, pacifiers and **nipple shields.**

3. The baby having a **tongue tie.**

4. **Late onset decreased milk supply** is fairly common in mothers attending our clinic and can cause late onset sore nipples. Why? When the milk flow slows, the baby tends to slip down on the nipple and/or pulls at the breast. **Watch this video** and how the baby pulls the nipple when the flow slows.

Infection of the nipples with Candida albicans ("thrush", "yeast")

It is vital that all health professionals understand that Candida **does not grow on normal skin**. I admit that though I knew this many years ago, even as a medical student, I didn't understand the connection and the importance of this fact to the problem of the mother having sore nipples. Thus, even if the mother has Candida growing on her nipples and/or there is a good reason to believe the mother's nipples are infected by Candida, Candida is *a secondary problem.* Candida is widely known in medicine as being "opportunistic", taking advantage of "weakness" in the immune system, so that people with cancer or AIDS, for example, are at risk of developing infection with Candida.

In the case of a breastfeeding mother, if Candida is causing infection of the nipples, and especially, if it is difficult to treat, or keeps returning after adequate treatment, there is an underlying problem. And that underlying problem is almost always damage to the nipple caused, almost always, by the baby's not latching on as well as he could. Once damage occurs, Candida takes the opportunity to grow there. And, to repeat, the damage is almost always due to a less than ideal latch. I repeat this because the emails I receive from breastfeeding mothers show that the mothers or health providers are fixated on the Candida and not the underlying problem.

There is no reason that Candida of the nipples could not be easily treated with our "all-purpose nipple ointment" (APNO) alone. So, if it is not easily treated, health providers should look for the underlying, *real* cause of sore nipples. The health provider should make sure the **baby's latch is good as it can be,** and not causing continuing damage to the nipple.

The "all-purpose nipple ointment" (APNO)

The APNO contains, usually, three ingredients, one that kills bacteria, one that kills Candida, and one that decreases inflammation. This combination essentially treats many, if not all, causes of nipple pain. Sometimes we will prescribe an APNO with an extra ingredient, ibuprofen powder, but we require this only rarely. Only rarely, because in our clinic we help the babies achieve a good latch as well as prescribe the ointment for the mother. The ointment should be seen as a *stop gap* measure only, something to give the mother relief until the underlying cause, a less than ideal latch, is treated.

Here is the recipe and the way I write a prescription:

1. Mupirocin ointment 2% (an antibiotic): 15 grams

2. Betamethasone ointment 0.1% (a corticosteroid): 15 grams

3. To which is added miconazole powder to a concentration of 2% miconazole

Total: 30 grams combined.

Apply sparingly after each feeding. Do not wash or wipe off.

Here are several notes on the APNO

1. Some health providers make up their own ointment or cream and call it APNO. That's fine, the terms "all-purpose nipple ointment" and APNO are not under copyright. But often the changes that are made in the "APNO" don't make sense and decrease its effectiveness. We have used this recipe for APNO for at least 25 years and its effectiveness has been proved by years of experience and patient follow-up. But, for example, the health provider prescribes creams instead of ointments, and we believe that creams are less effective. Or the health provider adds miconazole or clotrimazole cream instead of using the miconazole powder. If the APNO looks and feels like Vaseline, it might be the correct recipe. If it looks "creamy white" it is almost surely not our APNO.

2. In the United Kingdom and several other countries, miconazole powder is difficult to find, and most pharmacies don't seem to carry it. In that case, rather than substitute something, it is better just to use the first two ingredients, mupirocin and betamethasone. The mupirocin kills bacteria which

inhabit the areas of nipple damage, which may be microscopic and impossible to see with the naked eye, and the betamethasone treats the inflammation which is a large part of the pain the mother feels.

3. Mothers are commonly told to stop using the APNO after a week or two because, it seems, everyone is afraid the mother will get thinning of the skin of the nipples and areolas. We have *never* seen this happen in our clinic patients, but maybe that is due to our *not* using the APNO as the definite treatment. It is a **stop gap** treatment only. The answer to sore nipples is to **improve the way the baby latches on**. So, the mother uses the APNO until she doesn't need it, which is usually less than 1 or 2 weeks if we see the mother early and can help the mother latch the baby on well.

4. Many pharmacists, especially in hospital practice, get all in a rage because they feel that mupirocin should not be used. They argue that it is one of the few antibiotics still effective against methicillin resistant Staphylococcus aureus (MRSA), and we should not use it too much for fear that MRSA will become resistant to this drug as well. Well, bacterial overgrowth and infection of the nipples are often due to *Staphylococcus aureus*. So, we need a good antibacterial agent in the APNO.

This speaks volumes about how breastfeeding and breastfeeding mothers are seen in our society. Mothers' pain is not believed to be a real problem. Breastfeeding is nice but not necessary, so if the mother stops breastfeeding because of pain, well, that's not a great loss. Here we have a treatment, the APNO, that can decrease severe pain. But we cannot use it for a "trivial" problem like sore nipples. It makes us angry.

5. Many mothers are told to use the ointment only once or twice a day, or to wash or wipe it off before the baby goes back to the breast. No, we don't agree. Washing the nipples can cause them to dry out and make the pain worse. Wiping the ointment off is of no use. Our approach, as above? Apply sparingly after each feeding. Do not wash or wipe off.

6. It is necessary to say that **we do not make a cent** on the "all-purpose nipple ointment". We recommend it, not because we make money on it, which we

don't, but rather, **because it works,** and it often helps the mother manage until the baby's latch improves.

Other causes of sore nipples

1. Some dermatological problems can affect the nipples. These include eczema (atopic dermatitis) and psoriasis which seem the most common in our experience. **Treatment for these problems is the same as it would be in other parts of the body.** Mothers should not be told to interrupt breastfeeding to use such treatments.

2. **Vasospasm,** also can cause severe nipple and breast pain. It is often also called Raynaud's phenomenon. Vasospasm typically occurs after the baby comes off the breast and the temperature around the nipple falls from the warmth inside the baby's mouth to the cooler outside air. The nipple typically turns white from blood not reaching the end of the nipple and the mother often complains of a burning pain in the nipple. Sometimes this pain may radiate into the breast, so the mother may believe something is wrong in the breast itself. This is also called referred pain or radiating pain.

When the blood returns to the nipple, the mother may then feel a pulsating pain synchronized with the heart beat. Vasospasm is usually secondary to some other cause of pain in the nipples (the pain of a **less than adequate latch**), but sometimes may occur without any pain during latching on or during the feeding. Thus, in general, improving the latch and using the APNO will result in the vasospasm improving. However, it may take a week or two to disappear completely even after the mother has no pain with latching on or during the feeding. If the pain of vasospasm is severe, we will usually treat with oral **nifedipine**, slow release, 30 mg once a day. The dose of nifedipine can be increased to 30 mg of the slow release twice or even three times a day, but this is only very occasionally necessary. Sometimes the 30 mg once a day works very well, but when the mother stops the nifedipine, the pain returns. There is no reason to limit the time the mother is on the nifedipine, if it is necessary to alleviate her pain.

In this video, the baby has just come off the breast. The mother's nipple which was initially pink, turned white before our eyes. This blanching of the nipple was due constriction of the vessels to the nipple, causing the mother a burning pain. As time went on, the nipple returned to pink during which time the mother had a throbbing type of pain. Not all vasospasm hurts in exactly this way. For example, the pain on returning of blood to the nipple may not be throbbing and may even be absent.

3. A similar but somewhat different condition is called **mammary constriction syndrome.**

When the mother's nipples are cracked

Unfortunately, too often we see mothers only once the problems have gone very far, when the nipples have dramatic, wide-open cracks or craters.

In such cases, we have been trying and working with many treatments, most of which have been disappointing. In the last couple of years, we have found Medi-Honey (trademark) wound gel to be most helpful, but not in all cases either. The mother applies it inside the crack or crater once or twice a day and then applies the "all-purpose nipple ointment" over it and the rest of the areola. It is best to help mothers with sore nipples *early* before cracks result. But even when the nipples are cracked, **improving the latch** may improve the pain and result in healing of the nipples.

Some common solutions that should not be used:

1. Taking the baby off the breast "to rest the nipple(s)"

The most important treatment for sore nipples is, of course, prevention, helping the baby get **the best latch possible,** as soon as possible after the birth, which also helps the baby get more milk.

But if the mother already has sore nipples, the approach is not to take the baby off the breast. **The first step is to help the baby latch on well** and if necessary, use the "all-purpose nipple ointment". This approach works, so why are so many mothers not offered it?

Unfortunately, many of our clinic patients have been told to take the baby off the breast "to rest the nipples" on day 2 or 3 after birth. It is fair to ask this question: has everything *really* been tried to help this mother and baby before she was told to take the baby off the breast? It seems very unlikely.

There are many things to keep in mind as reasons for not taking the baby off the breast:

If the baby is taken off the breast, the real cause of the sore nipples (the latch) has not been dealt with. In fact, the baby, while off the breast, learns how to "latch" onto something quite different from the breast and when (and IF – a big "if") the baby goes back to the breast, the baby's latch could easily be even worse than it was initially.

A baby being fed away from the breast may mean the baby may **not go back to the breast.** As well, the baby being off the breast will likely decrease the mother's milk supply even if she expresses her milk diligently and the decrease in milk flow might consequently contribute to sore nipples again.

2. Nipple shields to "treat" sore nipples

We believe that using a **nipple shield** to treat sore nipples is even worse than taking the baby off the breast, though *neither* is a good solution. A nipple shield is very likely to result in a **significant decrease in milk supply.** And when the milk supply decreases, it becomes even more difficult to treat sore nipples. Additionally, a baby on a nipple shield is not truly latched on. A baby on a nipple shield has, essentially, been take off the breast. Thus, the baby's latch after being on a nipple shield and then being put back to the breast will be far from the ideal and may result in sore nipples again. Getting the baby to take a "bare" breast without a nipple shield after using the nipple shield for several days does not work easily for most mothers.

WHEN IT HURTS TO BREASTFEED PART 2

Breast or nipple pain in a breastfeeding mother is *never* normal nor should it be dismissed as insignificant or not worth looking into. Breast and nipple pain have a cause – most frequently related to the way the baby latches on to the breast – it should be investigated and treated appropriately.

See previous chapter on **nipple pain.**

Many physicians will consider any pain in the breast(s) of a breastfeeding mother to be mastitis. It is simply not true that pain in the breast means "mastitis". There are several causes for sore breasts and treatment with antibiotics will not improve most of them.

Sore breasts

What causes pain in the breast(s)?

Referred pain or radiating pain

A common cause of pain in the breast is what is generally called referred pain or also radiating pain. Referred pain describes a pain whose origin is *elsewhere* than where it is felt – in the case of a breastfeeding mother, the source of breast pain comes from **pain in the nipple**. How this happens is the same as for a person having angina (pain in the chest due to diminished blood flow to the heart) to feel pain not only in the area of the heart, but also in the arm and even down to the hand, though obviously the pain in the arm is not due to something wrong in the arm. In fact, it is possible that such pain is felt *only* in the arm and hand.

Another example of referred pain is seen in pregnant women who often have reflux of stomach acid into the esophagus (heartburn), but they may feel pain only in the neck.

Thus **pain from the nipple** *may* be felt in the breast and sometimes *only* in the breast once the nipple pain has diminished during the feeding or once the baby has come off the breast. This could be an example of referred pain or *radiating* pain. But it is not the only cause.

Vasospasm

Vasospasm, often called Raynaud's phenomenon, can be another cause of referred pain and can usually be felt in the nipple once the baby has come off the breast and the temperature of the nipple decreases; after the baby is off the breast, the nipple turns white from decreased blood flow to the nipple and subsequently back to its original colour once the blood vessels dilate again. It is usually secondary to nipple trauma. Mothers who have Raynaud's phenomenon when not pregnant or breastfeeding, do not *seem* to have a higher incidence of vasospasm of the nipple. Or, put another way, the vast majority of our patients with typical vasospasm do not give a history of vasospasm when they were not breastfeeding. The cause of vasospasm needs to be investigated and dealt with, which most often involves **correcting the latch**, and checking the baby for a possible **tongue tie**, a tongue tie being a cause of a less than ideal latch. The use of the "all-purpose nipple ointment" can help considerably until more definitive corrective measures are instituted. **Watch our video** on www.ibconline.ca of what a vasospasm looks like.

In the video, *the baby has just come off the breast. The mother's nipple which was initially pink, turned white before our eyes. This blanching of the nipple was due constriction of the vessels to the nipple, causing the mother pain, a burning pain. As time went on, the nipple returned to pink during which time the mother had a throbbing type of pain. Not all vasospasm hurts in exactly this way. For example, the pain on returning of blood to the nipple may not be throbbing and may even be absent.*

Milk Blisters can also cause pain that radiates into the breast and the white bleb on the nipple can go unnoticed or be ignored.

In all these cases, **adjusting the latch** and treating the nipples with the "all-purpose nipple ointment", will result in the breast pain diminishing as well.

95

Sore breasts within days of birth

Painful Engorgement

We do not accept that painful engorgement on the third or fourth day after birth is "normal" or even a good thing because "it means you are making lots of milk". We just don't believe this based on our long experience with mothers who just gave birth. We think that painful engorgement, anything more than fullness of the breast, is not normal and should not be considered normal or good. Sometimes the swelling of the breasts is so severe and so painful that mothers will decide not to breastfeed. And that is unfortunate because the problem is both preventable and treatable if it does occur.

Why do mothers have such severe engorgement? Basically, because the baby was *not* breastfeeding well during the first few days, not latched on well enough so that the breast drains as the baby breastfeeds.

Prevention of such painful engorgement depends on getting the baby to **latch on well** as soon as possible after birth. This approach starts with not giving the mother unnecessary intravenous fluids during labour and birth. Making the **breast crawl *routine* after birth**, allowing the baby to "climb" up to the breast while skin to skin with the mother immediately after birth would prevent multiple breastfeeding problems. A baby not affected by the **drugs given to the mother during labour and birth** and placed naked on the mother's chest will spontaneously crawl to the breast and latch on without help if given enough time (at least an hour, though many will latch on well before an hour). This is important as a start to breastfeeding and would help prevent a lot of breastfeeding problems in the first few days and after.

Breast and nipple pain in the first days after birth

Mothers, especially first time mothers, but not only first time mothers, need good information and support in the first few days to make sure the baby is **latched on well**. And **mothers need help especially** when they say their nipples

96

hurt. Hospital staff must not accept that it is "normal" for breastfeeding to hurt and pain should not be ignored even on day one.

When mothers complain about pain, the baby should not be removed from the breast and re-latched over and over again. Einstein apparently denied ever saying that "Madness is doing the same thing over and over and expecting a different result". But from the point of view of latching on, it's something worth remembering. Re-latching, removing the baby from the breast and re-latching yet again results in the mother's experiencing several painful latches instead of just one.

Often the baby's latch can be improved by putting some downward pressure on the baby's chin to open the mouth wider and/or shifting the baby so he is on the breast more asymmetrically which can be done without taking the baby off the breast. This is achieved by the mother's pushing the baby's bottom (bum, butt) into her chest with her forearm, while the baby is still latched on. The baby's latch becomes more asymmetric.

The baby can also be brought closer to the breast so that the latch is not "shallow". Increasing the flow of milk to the baby can go a long way in improving breast and nipple pain because **increased milk flow contributes to improving the latch**. And **breast compression** can help as well by increasing the flow of milk to the baby. A good latch improves milk flow to the baby; but a good milk flow also improves the baby's latch (a "virtuous" circle).

Go to www.ibconline.ca to watch videos showing babies drinking from the breast or not.

Even at this early stage, the mother could use our **"all-purpose nipple ointment"** to help her with the pain until the latch is improved.

If the pain is intolerable, pain medication such as ibuprofen can be used to help the mother continue breastfeeding while resolving and treating the cause of the pain.

Swaddling the baby, not looking for early cues that the baby is ready to feed

In many hospitals, and perhaps even with babies born at home, babies are often swaddled so that they don't wake up as frequently as they normally would if they were not swaddled. Swaddling has been shown to be harmful; it is the opposite of what babies need – which is skin to skin contact. Many studies, **here are just a few**, over the years have documented the value of skin to skin contact for premature babies, as well as full term, well and sick babies. Swaddled babies are, in fact, babies that are *separated from their mothers by layers of cloth* and are thus unaware of the regulation and signals provided by the mother's body. Swaddled babies sleep longer than is physiological, they spend much more energy trying to regulate their temperatures, they take longer to make their readiness to feed noticed, and unnoticed feeding cues may result in the babies not feeding as often as they would want or what is good for establishing breastfeeding. The same goes for use of the pacifier which causes the baby's feeding to be delayed and his feeding cues to go unnoticed.

Go to www.ibconline.ca to watch a video of *a baby who was so heavily swaddled that he did not show signs of wanting to feed. The mother was convinced that he had breastfed very well. But **when he was unswaddled**, he showed he was not satiated, that he wanted to feed more and he readily went to the breast and breastfed very well. Though the latch could be better, he is drinking a lot of milk, as can be seen by the long pauses in his chin.*

The consequences of the baby not feeding as frequently or as well as he would need, may result in painful breast engorgement for the mother on the third or fourth day when the milk production increases (milk "comes in". And, in yet another vicious circle, engorgement may make it difficult for the baby to latch on well.

How to prevent painful engorgement?

1. Ask the anaesthetist to avoid **large amounts of intravenous fluids** unless absolutely necessary. The large fluid volumes the mothers receive

routinely are hardly ever necessary and could be reduced significantly or avoided entirely. An intravenous line can be put up, but only enough fluid given to keep the vein open.

2. Have the baby skin to skin on the mother's chest immediately after birth and allow the baby time to crawl to the breast and latch on without help. Give sufficient time for the **breast crawl to be accomplished** and do not separate the mother and the baby.

3. **Get the best latch possible** as soon as possible after the birth.

4. Help the baby get more milk from the breast **using breast compression.**

5. Avoid bottles. If the baby truly needs supplements, which should be a rare situation, **a lactation aid at the breast** is a better way than to give bottles. And finger feeding to supplement is not a good method as it can be slow and arduous, and the baby is not on the breast. In fact, any supplementation off the breast should be avoided.

6. **A nipple shield** is not the answer to breastfeeding problems, including sore nipples and **baby not latching on** and only leads to poor drainage of the breast. And thus, not a way to prevent or treat engorgement.

7. If the mother and baby are leaving hospital within 24 hours as is now common, the parents need to know how to get good hands on help quickly. But if they need good hands on help quickly on leaving the hospital, they needed good hands on help while still in hospital. And if good hands on help is available in hospital, discharge should be delayed.

Blebs or blisters/blocked ducts/mastitis and on occasion, abscess

These problems almost always occur when the mother has a very good or even an abundant milk supply, but the baby does not have a good latch. And why does the baby not latch on well?

Because of:

99

1. How the baby is positioned and latched on

2. **Use of artificial nipples** such as bottles and **nipple shields** and pacifiers.

3. The baby has a tongue tie. Some tongue ties are obvious, but many tongue ties are more subtle and require an evaluation that goes farther than just looking and includes feeling under the baby's tongue as well and knowing what to feel for, especially how upward mobile the tongue is. Unfortunately, few health professionals, including lactation consultants, know how to evaluate whether or not the baby has a tongue tie.

Denial of tongue tie even being a possibility in breastfeeding problems has become a new battleground of breastfeeding. In some hospitals, pediatricians have taken the unbelievable step of forbidding nurses and lactation consultants, on pain of dismissal, of even mentioning to the parents that the baby may have a tongue tie. Oh, Galileo, who would have imagined that "scientists" in the 21st century would have such closed minds!

4.**The mother has had a** decrease in her milk supply. Though a less than adequate latch accompanying an abundant milk supply may cause the above mentioned problems, blebs or blisters/blocked ducts/mastitis may *also* occur because **milk supply has decreased.** Furthermore, recurrent blocked ducts may actually result in milk supply decreasing. **Late onset decreased milk supply** is not uncommon in the population of mothers experiencing breastfeeding problems and results the baby slipping down on the nipple, which hurts, and pulling at the breast which also hurts. The baby may pull off the breast when milk flow slows resulting in a breast that is not well drained.
In fact, the mother may feel her milk supply is still good, even "overabundant" because the breasts are frequently "full" even painfully so, after a feeding is over. "Full breasts" after a feeding strongly suggest that the breasts are not being drained properly, usually because of the baby's less than ideal latch. Watch these videos on www.ibconline.ca **Really good drinking with English text, Twelve day old nibbling, English Text**, **"Borderline" drinking** showing babies drinking well at the breast, or not. Watch the videos, read the texts and then watch the videos again.

100

Okay, that's how blocked ducts and mastitis and breast abscess are prevented, but how do I deal with these problems if I have them right now?

We believe that a blocked duct and mastitis are essentially the same condition, really only different degrees in the severity of the same condition. The same process seems to be happening in both, but on a different scale. The mother has an abundant milk supply or a milk supply that was once abundant and has now started to decrease in combination with the baby who is not latched on as well as he could be. Consequently, there is a part of the breast from which breastmilk is not draining as well as it should be. The milk being collected in a particular area of the breast results in swelling and the surrounding tissue being under pressure which results in inflammation of differing severity.

In any case, blocked ducts and mastitis often will get better without antibiotics. The mother should continue breastfeeding on the side affected, though sometimes the baby will not latch on, because of the swelling and the difficulty to latch on and because of the decrease in milk flow. The mother should get help with latching the baby on.

Sometimes the mother will have such pain that she cannot bear to put the baby on the breast. In such a case, pain medication such as ibuprofen or other non-steroidal **anti-inflammatory drugs**, can be used to provide pain relief and help the mother continue breastfeeding. Continuing breastfeeding will ultimately contribute to the mother's symptoms resolving sooner. **Improving the latch** is a way to prevent recurring blocked ducts or mastitis.

As much rest and sleep as possible is very helpful in this situation though new mothers often do not get as much rest as they would like and so they should ask for help in order to get some rest.

Often mothers with blocked ducts or mastitis have sore nipples at the same time and the **sore nipples** should be addressed as well.

What about antibiotics?

Even when the mother clearly has mastitis, with a painful lump in the breast, with redness of part of the breast, and the mother has fever, we will recommend caution with the antibiotics, partly because they are often not necessary and too often mothers are told that they must interrupt breastfeeding if they take antibiotics. **Not true.** We know of no antibiotic that requires a mother to interrupt breastfeeding.

If the mother has the symptoms of mastitis for less than 24 hours, we will give her a prescription for antibiotics, but ask her to wait before starting to take them. If the symptoms are obviously worsening over the next 12 or so hours, the mother should start the antibiotics. If the symptoms are improving or stable, we will ask her to wait another 12 hours and see. Often the mother will get better without antibiotics. If there is doubt about the situation, she should start the antibiotics.

If the mother has already had symptoms for 24 or more hours without the symptoms improving, she should start the antibiotics.

There is nothing magical about these times. They are only a guideline and each mother needs to be treated (or not), according to her own individual situation. Antibiotics for mastitis should be chosen based on the fact that mastitis is almost always caused by *Staphylococcus aureus*, which is *resistant almost* always to antibiotics such as amoxicillin, penicillin and erythromycin. If a mother's mastitis improves on amoxicillin, chances are her mastitis would have improved just as quickly without amoxicillin.

When mastitis is not getting any better at all within 24 hours of starting *appropriate* antibiotics, the mother may have Methicillin Resistant Staphylococcus Aureus (MRSA) and an antibiotic which works for MRSA should be started instead of the one she is on. Cotrimoxazole, which is a combination of two very different antibiotics, Trimethoprim/sulfamethoxazole (TMP/SMX), and thus, more likely to be effective against *Staphylococcus aureus*.

How quickly should the mastitis improve? Usually mastitis starts to get better over 24 to 48 hours, whether the mother is on antibiotics or not. Pain and fever are decreasing, and within 2 to 3 days the mother is starting to feel better. The lump in the breast may take a week or more to resolve completely, but by day 3 or 4 should be getting progressively smaller and less tender.

Breast abscess

Mastitis that does not follow the improvement as above or seems to improve but not completely could be an **abscess**. If an abscess is present, on examination, one can often tell that there is fluid in the lump, and that fluid, in the context of a mastitis not improving, is likely to be pus and the mother has an abscess. However, a blocked duct sometimes, we believe, then turns into a galactocoele, also called a milk cyst.

Surgeons like to operate. It's "their thing". But operating on a **lactating breast** is fraught with possible complications. There is a better way of treating a breast abscess than making incisions in the breast. Intervention radiologists have a better approach.

Breast lumps that are not any of the above

There are many types of lumps in the breast that do not fit the clinical picture of any of the above problems. Breast cancer usually is not painful in the early stages. The issue for the breastfeeding mother and her doctor is how to deal with a lump that may require **further investigation**. It is best to avoid surgery on the lactating breast if it is at all practical and possible. Usually, it is possible.

LOW BLOOD SUGAR AND BREASTFEEDING

There are two measures that can and should be introduced into routine hospital practices after birth, the absence of which, in the vast majority of hospitals, is causing many mothers to stop breastfeeding even though they had originally intended to breastfeed.

Skin to skin contact helps maintain a newborn's blood sugar

First, babies should be skin to skin with their mothers immediately after birth, not only **premature babies** but **all babies**. Even many babies who are showing signs of difficulty adjusting to the outside environment, *especially* these babies, often will adapt better to their new environment if placed skin to skin with the mother. Skin to skin contact between the mother and baby should be considered both normal and at the same time, a therapeutic measure. Skin to skin contact should be the *standard of care* to improve a baby's adaptation to the outside environment. It is proved that a baby who is skin to skin with his mother maintains blood sugar levels better than a baby who is not or who is in an incubator. Skin to skin contact, without the baby being dressed, obviously, should be routine postpartum care for *at least* the first few hours after birth. (We know that it is obvious that the baby should not be dressed in skin to skin contact, but we have seen photos of babies supposedly "skin to skin" who are completely dressed).

Not only does the baby maintain his blood sugar better, but also, is much more stable with regard to his heart rate, respiratory rate and blood pressure.

Table 4 Metabolic, circulatory and respiratory adaptation of the infants at 90 min postpartum.

	Skin-to-skin group (n = 25)	Cot group (n = 25)	p value
Heart rate/min	136.6 ± 6.9	140.7 ± 9.0	ns
Resp. rate/min	44.3 ± 7.9	49.8 ± 10.2	0.05
Skin colour: pink	25	25	
Blood glucose (mmol/l)	3.17 ± 0.7	2.56 ± 0.71	0.001
pH	7.32 ± 0.04	7.32 ± 0.06	ns
Δ Base excess (mmol/l) (difference between values in cord blood and in sample at 90 min postpartum)	3.4 ± 2.7	1.8 ± 2.6	0.05

ns = Not significant.

*Skin to skin contact immediately after birth helps maintain
the newborn baby's blood sugar and other functions. From
Christensson K, Siles C,
Morena L, Belaustequi A, de la Fuente P,
Lagercrantz H, et al. Temperature, metabolic
adaptation and crying in healthy full-term
newborns cared for skin-to-skin or in a cot*
Acta Paediatr 1992;81:488–93

As well, skin to skin contact immediately after birth provides an opportunity for babies to start breastfeeding and getting breastmilk from the breast very soon after birth. Breastmilk is a very good way to help maintain blood sugar levels in the baby, **better than formula.**

Secondly, mothers should be shown how to know whether their baby is receiving breastmilk from the breast – that is, to be able to tell whether the baby is *drinking* milk well or not. If the baby is drinking well, the mother should be re-assured; if the baby is not drinking well, then the first step to take is to **improve the breastfeeding** and help the baby **get more milk from the breast.**

Hypoglycemia (low blood sugar) is one of the commonest reasons for formula supplementation in the first few days after birth. **But most babies are tested for low blood sugar for no good reason, and most babies get formula by bottle also unnecessarily.**

1. Doing routine blood sugars on *every* baby at birth is another example of how "worrying about being sued" causes damage to babies and creates unnecessary anxiety in the parents and results in unnecessary "treatment". Many hospitals in the US have this policy of doing a blood sugar at birth on *every baby,* whether or not there is a reason, and more and more are adopting this policy in Canada. Interestingly, most pediatricians and neonatologists don't seem to know what normal is. They look at a number and say, "give formula".

2. In fact, nobody agrees on what is a normal blood sugar in newborns. Everyone has a different number they consider "too low".

3. The blood sugar in babies is more or less the same as the mother's blood sugar at birth and then over the next 1 to 2 hours the sugar drops, *normally.* For some babies, the glucose drops *normally* into the range many would call "too low". But this drop in the blood sugar is NORMAL! (see the graph). And the blood sugar rises again over the following hour or two *even if the baby is not fed.* This has been shown not only in humans but also in all mammals that have been studied. Treating "low blood sugar" in this circumstance is treating NORMAL and thousands of babies across North America are being unnecessarily supplemented with formula for what is, in fact, a normal blood sugar.

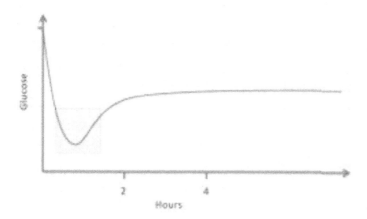

Normal glucose levels in normal newborns in the
first hours after birth

Various physicians have become unnerved because the above graph does not
contain units of blood or plasma glucose. That's not the point. The point is that
it is normal for the blood sugar to drop in the first hour or two after birth. You
want graphs with numbers? Here is a **study from 1986** and still after more
than 30 years, many pediatricians don't know about the drop. Here is **another
study from 2000**. And here is an **article from a world expert** on the issue of
hypoglycemia. What does Dr Jane Hawdon write in this article?

"Almost all babies have a sharp fall in blood glucose in hours after birth and
then a slow rise from a nadir which occurs in the first 12 h... However as with
other potentially precarious postnatal adaptations, there is a backup plan and
the healthy baby responds to falls in blood glucose by mobilising and using
alternative fuels to glucose. Thus, healthy babies are unlikely to manifest
clinical signs or sustain brain injury during this physiological postnatal fall of
blood glucose."

4. Separation of the mother and baby causes blood sugar to drop further and
skin to skin contact with the mother helps maintain blood sugar levels in the

baby. Skin to skin contact also affords the baby an opportunity to feed at the breast.

5. The mother's own colostrum is what the baby is meant to get and banked breastmilk can be used in addition to mother's breastmilk if necessary to prevent and treat low blood sugar in newborn babies. This is because breastmilk does not stimulate the **production of insulin** in the baby as much as does formula. For this reason, we recommend that mothers whose babies are at high risk for low blood sugar **express and store their milk** starting at 35 to 36 weeks gestation so the baby, if necessary, can receive colostrum instead of formula. There is no evidence that hand expression of milk at this stage increases the risk of premature birth. See the photo below that shows the amount of colostrum one mother expressed before the baby was born.

6. There is evidence that babies who are at risk for low blood sugar and are fed at the breast immediately after birth are **less likely to become clinically hypoglycemic and actually have higher blood sugars than babies fed formula as their first feeding.**

7. There is no evidence that **a baby who is born big** (some hospital policies say 4 kg=8lb 12oz or higher) is at risk for low blood sugar even if his mother is *not* diabetic. On the contrary, such babies are at lower risk of hypoglycemia because they have lots of body fat that can be broken down into compounds called ketone bodies.

8. **Ketone bodies** protect the baby's brain from the effects of low blood sugar and ketone bodies are present in much higher concentrations in the blood of babies breastfed (or fed colostrum or breastmilk) than in the blood of babies formula fed. Babies fed both breastmilk and formula have a lower but intermediate response.

9. There is no need for babies at risk for low blood sugar (infants of diabetic mothers, both type 1 and type 2) to automatically go to special care. They should stay with the mother, skin to skin, be fed on demand and get help from the nursing staff to make sure the baby feeds well at the breast. Pre-expressed colostrum can be fed by spoon, open cup or, preferably, **lactation aid at the**

108

breast. See this article on **mothers with gestational diabetes** and **this article on mothers with type 1 diabetes,** where the authors felt that mothers and baby should be kept together and the babies not necessarily sent to special care. In the article on mothers with gestational diabetes, the authors write: "breastfed infants had a significantly higher mean blood glucose level compared to those who were formula fed for their first feed".

10. Bottom line? There is a lot of *hysteroglycemia* out there and the "treatment" of it is causing many babies to be unnecessarily supplemented with formula, most often with bottles. In one case of a mother who contacted us, the baby was admitted to the NICU because an unnecessary blood sugar was done shortly after birth (during the time that the blood sugar sometimes NORMALLY drops to "hypoglycemic" levels.) The baby had an intravenous with glucose and also was given formula, by bottle, of course. The mother was feeding with a **nipple shield** (for reasons that did not seem clear, probably because the baby refused the breast after receiving bottles, but to me NO reason for nipple shield use is clear) and pumping her breasts. The baby was in the NICU for several days at great cost to the health system. All because of an unnecessary blood sugar being done as a "routine". This baby had no risk factors for hypoglycemia. In another recent case, a baby whose mother did have gestation diabetes was "ripped from her breast" as she said, so that the baby's blood sugar could be measured. The baby was then transferred to NICU even though, apparently, the baby had been breastfeeding well.

BREASTFEEDING, BILIRUBIN AND JAUNDICE

Jaundice in the first few days after birth

It is usual and normal for babies to become jaundiced in the first few days after birth. But the bilirubin that causes the yellow colour of the baby's skin is **protective, it's an antioxidant**. There is some recent evidence as well, that **bilirubin helps fight off infection**.

Too often, we treat higher than average bilirubin levels in a sort of panic state, and too often at the expense of breastfeeding. Hardly ever, it seems, does anyone routinely take time to watch babies **drinking at the breast** right after birth and *before* they become jaundiced. A baby who feeds well at the breast is not likely to have higher than average bilirubins. Even when the baby does have higher than average levels of bilirubin, improving the breastfeeding prevents the real issue of why the baby is jaundiced more than average: that is, poor breastfeeding. Once the jaundice becomes a worry for the staff on the ward, the solution almost always becomes phototherapy and very often formula feeding with bottles. This approach **misses the real issue which is**:

Here is the real issue: Is the baby breastfeeding well? Is the baby actually getting breastmilk from the breast or is the baby just holding the breast in his mouth and making sucking motions without drinking? **A baby is not getting breastmilk from the breast just because he has the breast in his mouth and makes sucking movements.** Knowing how to tell whether the baby is latched on well and actually getting breastmilk makes a difference to everything that should happen next. But it seems that all that matters is the bilirubin level.

If a jaundiced baby is not drinking well at the breast, that baby and the mother need help with breastfeeding. Supplementing of formula should be done only if **helping the mother with the latch** and using **breast compression** do not increase the intake of breastmilk by the baby. And supplementing with the mother's own expressed milk (the first choice), properly screened donor breastmilk (every hospital with maternity and pediatrics should have a

110

breastmilk bank), and formula (if necessary) should be done with **a lactation aid at the breast.**

If the baby is not getting milk directly from the breast, **how can the mother express milk that is "not there"?** The milk *is* there, in almost all cases. The baby is just not receiving the milk, usually because of a **poor latch.** Colostrum starts being produced at about 16 or 17 weeks gestation and accumulates during the pregnancy.

If the baby is not receiving milk from the breast, it is possible and desirable for the mother to express her milk (hand expression often works best) and feed it to the baby with a **lactation aid at the breast,** preferably, or with an open cup, or with a small spoon. But the mother should be receiving help all the time to get the baby to latch on well and receive the milk from the breast, with **breast compression** often helping the baby receive more milk.

It is normal for babies to have jaundice during the first few days of life, (though not usually on day 1. The bilirubin which causes the yellow colour of the baby's skin rises to a peak, usually on the third day of life and then decreases. It is called "physiologic jaundice" because it is normal. Where does the bilirubin come from?

Bilirubin is formed when old red blood cells die, and hemoglobin is released into the blood. The globin part of the hemoglobin is recycled leaving heme, which is toxic, and the body wants to get rid of it. So, the body breaks down the heme to salvage an iron molecule from it, and forms a compound called biliverdin. The biliverdin, in its turn, is transformed by an enzyme, called biliverdin reductase (for keen students of biochemistry) into bilirubin.

The usual, *normal* jaundice that occurs in newborns is due, at least partly, to the fact that the hemoglobin and thus the red blood cells of the fetus and newborn are different from that of the older child and adult and have a much shorter life span than the red blood cells of adults (80 days on average for the fetal hemoglobin containing cells compared to 120 days on average for the adult hemoglobin containing cells). Also, newborns have a lot of red blood cells, which they needed in utero, and thus, many more on average than an adult.

111

Bilirubin Metabolism

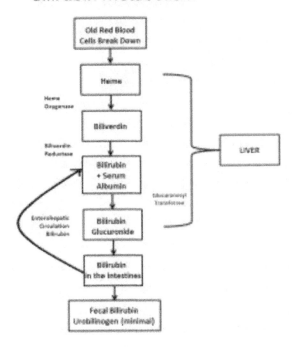

How bilirubin is formed from dying red blood cells

The body does not need to make bilirubin. Biliverdin, the step before the production of bilirubin, is easy to get rid of. Yet the body *does* make bilirubin and the body rarely does something without a good reason. Indeed, the energy cost to the body in order to make bilirubin from biliverdin is considerable. Every molecule of biliverdin that is converted to bilirubin uses up one molecule of NADPH, and for those of you who might actually remember the biochemistry you learned (or didn't) in school, that's a powerful lot of energy.

Bilirubin is an antioxidant and there is good evidence that mild to moderate levels of bilirubin helps protect our cells against oxidative stress. There is a fascinating association of higher than average levels of bilirubin in an inherited condition called Gilbert's syndrome (a condition that results in life long mild elevations of bilirubin) and a lower incidence of atherosclerosis, now believed to be an inflammatory disease. When people with Gilbert's syndrome get an infection or are stressed, their bilirubin goes up, again suggesting that bilirubin helps protect.

So how does this all fit with the problem of too high bilirubin in a 3 or 4 day old baby? When a breastfed baby has a higher than average bilirubin level, it *can* be and often is, a sign that the baby is not breastfeeding well.

The approach is to help the mother and baby breastfeed better, so the baby receives more milk from the breast, done by **improving the baby's latch**, by using **breast compressions**, giving the baby an opportunity to breastfeed more frequently and by switching breasts and if necessary, supplementing the baby with a **lactation aid at the breast**. The problem is not the bilirubin, *the problem is inadequate feeding*. The bilirubin is an "innocent bystander", blamed for brain damage when it is the dehydration, acidosis and other metabolic abnormalities that are the problem in severe cases of poor breastfeeding. Phototherapy may bring down the bilirubin, but it doesn't fix the *real* problem, which is that the baby is not breastfeeding well. Fix the breastfeeding before the situation deteriorates and **phototherapy, which may not be harmless**, and supplementation would not be necessary much of the time.

With regard to ABO incompatibility or other causes of incompatibility, if the baby is breastfeeding well, there is no reason for supplementation. Supplementing the breastfeeding implies that breastmilk causes jaundice. It doesn't. In the case of hemolysis, it's the rapid breakdown of red blood cells that is the problem, not breastmilk. If the baby is not breastfeeding well, the first thing to do is help the mother and baby with breastfeeding.

It is for this reason that the so called "breastmilk jaundice" (see the next chapter), which is seen in exclusively breastfed babies up to 3 or more months after birth is *not a problem* as most, or at least many, physicians seem to believe. If the baby is breastfeeding well, drinking well at the breast (**This baby is drinking very well at the breast**) and gaining weight well and there are no signs of liver problems (which causes another sort of jaundice), then

113

"breastmilk jaundice" is good, not bad, the bilirubin acting to protect the baby's cells.

SO-CALLED BREASTMILK JAUNDICE

So-called "breastmilk jaundice" is considered abnormal by many physicians, perhaps even the majority of physicians. Even those who understand that it is usually normal for exclusively breastfed, well gaining babies of 3 or 6 weeks of age and even older to have visually obvious jaundice, may, due to the general fear of jaundice, advise the mother to interrupt breastfeeding for 24 to 48 hours in order to "prove" that the "problem" is due to breastfeeding. I have been contacted by mothers who were told they needed to interrupt breastfeeding for a week, and occasionally even completely because of this "problem".

In fact, stopping breastfeeding and giving formula by bottle for even 24 to 48 hours can cause significant problems with breastfeeding, and stopping the breastfeeding for a week may mean stopping the breastfeeding altogether for that baby. Where the notion of stopping breastfeeding for a week comes from, is obvious. The idea is that stopping breastfeeding for 24 to 48 hours is to "prove the jaundice is due to breastmilk". But when a doctor says to a mother that she must stop for a week, the doctor is saying "Oh no, jaundice! Bilirubin is so dangerous! It will take a week to get rid of the jaundice."

It is typical of babies with "breastmilk jaundice" to be bursting with obvious good health. There is nothing in the baby's story of concern, no physical findings of concern and observation of the feeding shows a baby drinking very well at the breast. Though we do not generally recommend doing tests to rule out other causes of jaundice, because a healthy, growing baby, with no enlargement of the liver and clear colourless urine is unlikely to have a problem with his liver, we understand that others wish to do tests once to rule out liver disease.

On the other hand, a baby who is jaundiced because he is **not getting enough from the breast** may **remain jaundiced** into the second and even the third week of life, so one cannot simply assume that a baby of 2 or 3 weeks of age who is jaundiced has "breastmilk jaundice". Interestingly enough, most exclusively breastfed babies who are *not* getting enough from the breast are *not* jaundiced. And that may be because it is *normal* and good to have "breastmilk jaundice".

115

Why? Why might jaundice be good?

Because bilirubin is an **antioxidant**, a powerful cytoprotectant and **there is good evidence** that mild to moderate levels of bilirubin may protect the body against oxidative stress. A cytoprotectant protects cells from damage. There is evidence as well, that **bilirubin helps fight off infection**.

There is a fascinating association of higher than average levels of bilirubin in an inherited condition called **Gilbert's syndrome** and a lower incidence of atherosclerosis, now believed to be an inflammatory disease. This has been known for many years. One physician with whom I trained in 1970 had Gilbert's syndrome and he lorded it over us because he kept insisting his risk of myocardial infarction was much lower than ours. And he always looked as if he had a nice tan, 12 months of the year. In fact, people with Gilbert's are, apparently, otherwise normal. Frequently, the jaundice is not easily noticeable in such people, but with infection or stress, the bilirubin may rise. Interesting? Maybe bilirubin is a good thing after all, rising to protect the individual when she or he has an infection of some sort.

If there is any question that the baby may have liver disease, a serum bilirubin, testing for both indirect *and* direct levels of bilirubin should be done. It is usually easy enough to suspect liver disease causing jaundice. The baby's urine is often brownish, and the bowel movements are paler than usual, though this is not so easy to appreciate as an exclusively breastfed baby's bowel movements are normally paler than an adult's. The most common cause in a baby of 3 or 4 weeks of age is a condition called biliary atresia, where the ducts leading from the liver to the baby's intestinal tract are blocked. On physical examination by a physician or nurse practitioner, the liver is usually found to be enlarged, and the spleen is also often enlarged as well.

Case study

The baby in this photo is 7 weeks old. He was born slightly premature at 36 weeks gestation. Surprisingly he was exclusively breastfed in hospital, which would be unusual in most hospitals, where too often such a baby of 36 weeks gestation, in spite of no medical problems, would automatically receive formula. Why? Because such a baby is at risk of low blood sugar. Ah, no, that is not really true, **not if he is breastfeeding well**.

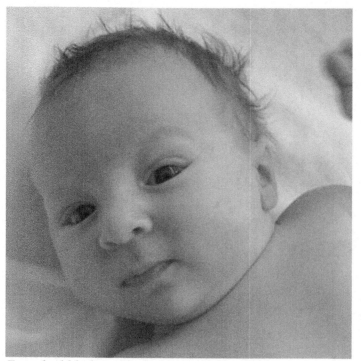

7 week old baby with obvious jaundice. He is Breastfeeding exclusively, receiving lots of milk from the breast and gaining weight well. His urine is clear like water, and there is no evidence of liver disease.

Here are his weights: At birth 2.87 kg (6lb 5oz). At 7 weeks when we first saw him, 4.57 kg (10lb 1oz). Certainly, all will agree that the weight gain is quite good.

So, what did we do?

We did not worry the mother by saying that the jaundice was a problem.

However, we did tell her that it was normal for many exclusively breastfed well gaining babies to be jaundiced so that if anyone did worry her about it she wouldn't worry (interestingly, the mother had not noticed the jaundice).

We did not do any blood tests, but we did ask about the colour of the urine and stool. The mother stated that the baby's urine was clear as water and the bowel movements looked normal. When we examined the baby, the baby's liver and spleen were not enlarged.

We did not tell her to interrupt breastfeeding and I urged her to continue *exclusive* breastfeeding.

We did help her to overcome her sore nipples. That was easy in this case, despite the baby being seen so late at the clinic, simply by helping her adjust **how the baby was latching on.**

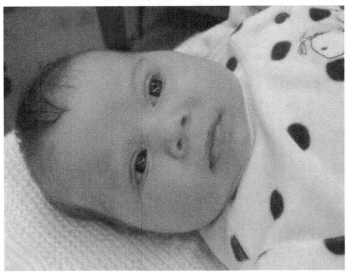

One month old baby with breastmilk jaundice. He is exclusively breastfeeding, gaining weight well, urine is clear as water, and there is no enlargement of the liver and spleen. There is no reason to interrupt breastfeeding. It is harmful to the baby to be taken off the breast and

118

given
formula as was recommended by the family doctor.

Unlike the previous baby in the first photo, this baby's mother was under pressure to stop breastfeeding both from the baby's doctor and from the mother's family. There was no reason to stop breastfeeding, even for one feeding.

And here a 16 day old with jaundice who is breastfeeding beautifully. Unfortunately, we did not manage to film this baby in time to show how well he was drinking. But he was drinking a lot of milk. Remember how to know a baby is drinking well (**pauses in the chin**).

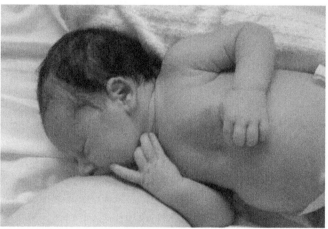

Sixteen day old baby with obvious jaundice.
Breastfeeding very well, receiving lots of milk from the
breast. There was no indication of liver disease. There
is no need and it is not good to interrupt breastfeeding.

So why not interrupt breastfeeding for 48 hours in the above babies?

Because it is not good practice and disrupts breastfeeding and the baby is exposed to risks of formula feeding.

It is definitely easier for the doctor with a formula=breastmilk mindset, true, but....

Not easier for the mother. It is easy to recommend that the mother express her milk while the baby is being fed formula, but not always easy for the mother to do so. Sometimes mothers become painfully engorged despite pumping.

Not easier for the baby. Here is a secret. Many babies do not respond well to formula. We don't hear much about the negative effects on babies drinking formula. For example, many vomit formulas. Some, even by 3 weeks of age will not drink from a bottle. And the baby loses out on the **relationship of breastfeeding** and is exposed to other risks connected with formula feeding.

May undermine the mother's confidence in breastfeeding and breastmilk. Mothers get messages from public health departments, from magazines, from their doctors that breastfeeding is very important. But when the baby has "breastmilk jaundice", "you need to stop breastfeeding and give formula, or your baby may be brain damaged". What's the message? Breastfeeding is dangerous.

May result in breastfeeding difficulties. The common myth amongst many health professionals that there is no problem with giving breastfed babies bottles. How can they think this if they have had any experience at all with breastfeeding and helping breastfeeding mothers? It can only come from the idea that breastfeeding and bottle feeding are the same. Of course, there is no lack of bottle makers flogging their "natural bottles" or bottles as "just like breastfeeding" but that's marketing and just not true. "Interrupting" breastfeeding carries an inherent danger of lowering the milk supply and the baby not latching on after being on bottles for a couple of days. Furthermore, some mothers stop breastfeeding as a result of the "interruption" because the baby, now, not as happy at the breast as he was, well, "might as well pump and give my milk by bottle".

May result in the mother thinking: "My milk is dangerous for the baby". Many doctors will use the "brain damage" card if the mother is reluctant to interrupt breastfeeding, but even pushing the mother to stop breastfeeding is enough to plant the seed in the mother's mind that breastfeeding is dangerous.

"My baby is getting all these tests done". Some mothers have stopped breastfeeding in order to stop the baby being stuck for blood every few days. And what information comes from these tests? Rarely, if ever, does the physician get any more information than the level of the bilirubin that day. And how does that change the situation? The result of such bilirubin tests is basically, "Hmmm, the bilirubin is still above a level I like to see. So, let's do another in a few days".

A sad case and a good question, the first from a mother's personal blog, the second from an email:

1. "My nipples looked like hamburger meat, yet I kept going. I wanted to succeed. Then his pediatrician told me he had breast milk jaundice. She gave me 3 cans of formula and told me to take him off breast milk for 3 days and feed him the formula instead. I was distraught. All I could think was *'I have gone through all of this to breast feed him and here I was **poisoning** him the entire time'* (our italics and bold emphasis). His jaundice cleared up in 2 days and I quit breastfeeding. I lost all control over my emotions in the parking lot of the doc's office and called my husband to tell him I will never breastfeed again for as long as I live."

   Comments: Well, if the mother's **nipples were sore**, then the baby did not have **a good latch**. This is not "maybe the baby had a poor latch". The baby definitely had a poor latch! And much could have been done to help the mother. In fact, **it's often very easy to help a mother with sore nipples,** *if one knows how.* But then what do most doctors know about helping mothers to latch on babies? Most know nothing.

   What did the pediatrician do to help this mother? Nothing, it seems. It sounds as if she did not even bother to refer her to someone who *could* help her. I guess this is yet another pediatrician who believes that it is normal to have sore nipples when breastfeeding. Does the pediatrician really believe that the fact that she is a pediatrician means that she cannot help the mother because "the baby is my patient, not the mother"? A breastfeeding mother and baby are a pair, a dyad, a couple, intimately connected to each other and because of

121

that, the mother is also the pediatrician's patient. The mother is the pediatrician's patient because this pediatrician probably learned only one thing in her training: Breast is best. So, if the mother stops breastfeeding, she is taking away from the baby the best feeding, which is breastfeeding. Many mothers with the sort of pain this mother had, would have quit well before she went to the pediatrician. She toughed it out because she really wanted to breastfeed. But "breastmilk jaundice" was the last straw, it seems.

As mentioned already in this article, "breastmilk jaundice" is not only *not bad* for the healthy well-breastfeeding baby, but actually is good. But "breastmilk jaundice" and three cans of formula sealed the fate of this mother's breastfeeding.

Furthermore, because of the poor latch, it is possible, even likely, that the baby actually was not getting enough milk and the problem was not "breastmilk jaundice" at all, but rather "not enough breastmilk jaundice".

And the pediatrician gave the mother 3 cans of formula? That is appalling. That is not help. And it's not a gift, because this mother will now spend a lot of money in the next months to pay for that "gift". Who gains? The formula company, of course, because chances are the mother will then go on to buy the same brand of formula for the entire time the baby is formula fed. By what right does this pediatrician become a marketing agent for formula?

What message did the mother receive from this simple exchange with the pediatrician? "I have gone through all of this to breast feed him and here I was *poisoning* him the entire time". Poisoning her baby with bilirubin! Well done doctor. And not surprisingly, she will not breastfeed any of her babies to come.

2. "I think it is a bit odd that the doctors were really adamant about feeding him every 3 hours in the hospital and making sure he was nursing really well before we went home and now they think that is what is making him sick. I guess what I am emailing you for is to see if I can get a clearer explanation for this and for my child's affliction."

My comments: Maybe these doctors are more supportive than the pediatrician in the previous case, but maybe not. Yes, they want to make sure the baby feeds well, a worthy goal. But they may be nervous and worried about breastfeeding working out because they don't know what to expect from breastfeeding and don't know **how to know a baby is getting milk**. As with many doctors and other health professionals, they believe in the numbers. But it's not how frequently a baby drinks, it's *how well* the baby drinks. A baby who drinks *well* 6 times a day is better off than a baby that drinks *poorly* 8 or 10 or 12 times a day. It is not true that a baby is drinking milk simply because he has the breast in his mouth and makes sucking motions. **How to know a baby is drinking well at the breast?**

Go to www.ibconline.ca to watch videos showing babies drinking from the breast or not.

And what message did the mother get from the doctors? That breastmilk makes your baby "sick". Not just sick, but the baby has an "affliction", a word of Biblical resonance. Something like the 11 plagues of Egypt: Blood, frogs, lice, jaundice...

FEED ON ONE BREAST OR BOTH?

Many mothers are now being advised to feed the baby on one breast at a feeding only, meaning that the baby should "finish" the whole feeding on the one breast and not be offered the other. Though the number who email us about breastfeeding problems varies from day to day, usually, on any given day about 1 in 4 of mothers experiencing breastfeeding problems are feeding the baby on just one breast at a feeding. Even some who are supplementing with bottles and formula are offering the baby only one breast at each feeding and then giving the bottle. This seems to underline how mothers and those who "help" her have lost touch with normal breastfeeding or never had a real understanding of breastfeeding and how it works.

This idea is presumably based on the information that the amount of fat in breastmilk increases as the baby drinks more milk from the breast, as this study International Breastfeeding Journal 2009;4:7-13, as well as several other studies suggest. This increase in fat as more milk is removed from the breast (by pumping) is likely to be true as well when the baby is on the breast and *drinking*. But this notion of feeding the baby on only one breast at each feeding, to follow a "rule", has resulted in many mothers running into difficulty with late onset decreased milk supply.

To emphasize, this idea of milk increasing in the concentration of fat as more milk is released from the breast depends on the baby drinking, not just sucking *without actually getting milk*. It is a myth, and important enough for me to repeat several times in these pages, that a baby is not necessarily getting milk simply because the baby is latched on and making sucking motions.

Moreover, all breastmilk the baby gets contains fat, even the very first milk the baby gets when he latches on. There is no such thing as "no-fat" breastmilk, though mothers are sometimes told by health providers that they are producing only "skimmed milk". That is absurd.

Is the baby drinking or not?

Go to www.ibconline.ca to watch videos showing babies drinking from the breast or not.

Rules and breastfeeding do not go together

In other words, it is not a good idea to feed the baby on just one side, *to follow a rule*. Yes, making sure the baby "finishes" the first side before offering the second can help treat poor weight gain or fussiness in the baby, but *rules and breastfeeding do not go together well*. How does the mother know that the baby is "finished" the first side? Because the baby does not drink much from the breast even with breast compression.

If the baby is not drinking, actually *receiving milk from the breast*, there is no point in just keeping the baby sucking without getting any milk for long periods of time. It is best to "finish" one side and then offer the other. The approach of feeding one side without "listening" to the baby often ends up with a decrease in milk supply.

In our video on www.ibconline.ca, *the baby tries to latch on, but the latch is not particularly good. He sucks, gets small amounts of milk, but pulls off and on the breast. He is "gassy", and not happy at the breast. But despite the almost universal belief that "gas" causes the baby to act like this or that gas causes the baby to be fussy and "colicky", gas causes none of this. This baby is acting like this due to* **late onset decreased milk supply** *and one-sided feedings.*

Many mothers will keep the baby on the first breast until the baby is deeply asleep. Thus, the baby may not take the second side even if offered it. Let us imagine that the baby drank 80%, say, of the milk he needed from the first side. If he remains on the breast until deeply asleep, he might not wake up to take the second side, not being particularly hungry at that point. The baby should be offered the second breast when he is not drinking much any longer even with breast compression, not when he's asleep.

Furthermore, babies tend to receive less milk in the late afternoon and evening than in the morning, so what might work in the early morning (baby finishing the feeding with one breast only) may not work in the late afternoon or evening. If the baby cries and fusses in the evening, the mother who has been advised "one breast/feeding" may keep putting the baby back to the same breast and finally conclude that she needs to give the baby a bottle of formula. And surprise, surprise, the baby is satisfied and sleeps 3 hours or even longer. The mother may even be convinced that she does not produce enough milk. That evening bottle, if given regularly, is also likely to lead to decreased milk flow and as the milk supply continues to decrease, the problem may get worse and worse. Even if the mother puts previously expressed milk into the evening bottle, that does not prevent the problem.

Most mothers tend to have less milk in the late afternoons and evenings. One thing that works is for the mother to lie down with the baby and feed the baby side to side. Babies that fuss when the mother feeds the baby sitting up tend to be less fussy when they are feeding lying down side by side. The baby will often fall asleep and so will the mother sometimes.

Formula companies know the effects of substituting a bottle in the late afternoon or evening on the milk supply. Most formula company "information pamphlets" emphasize "giving the father a chance to feed the baby". And the time for the father to do this? In the late evening or night, so that the mother "can rest".

On top of everything else, what may work when the baby is a month of age, say, may not work when the baby is 3 or 4 months old. Yet, if the mother continues to believe that one breast at each feeding is best, the milk supply will continue to decrease, and many symptoms of late onset decreased milk supply may occur.

The symptoms of late onset decreased milk supply include:

1. Decreased weight gain or even weight loss. On the other hand, many babies will continue to gain weight reasonably well in spite of a decreased milk supply and flow to the baby. This problem, usually, is the problem of the mother who started off with an abundant milk supply and often the milk supply is still fairly good. But the baby's behaviour shows that something is wrong. The real issue is not weight gain or whether the baby is getting enough milk "a baby

126

should get at his age", but the baby's behaviour at the breast. The following are 3 frequently made, but *incorrect*, diagnoses:

- "colic" and general fussiness with the baby pulling at the breast, letting go of the breast and coming back to the breast and pulling off the breast again. Babies who cry a lot are usually crying a lot because they want more milk, not because they have "colic". And they may want more milk *even if they are continuing to gain weight well.*

- "reflux" with the baby pulling at the breast, letting go of the breast and coming back to the breast and pulling off the breast again. We believe that "reflux" is very uncommon in exclusively breastfed babies.

- "allergy to something in the mother's milk" with the baby pulling at the breast, letting go of the breast and coming back to the breast and pulling off again, and not rarely having blood in the bowel movements.
2. The baby starts to suck his fingers much of the time. This is important because this may be the only other symptom associated with late onset decreased milk supply. So, the baby is generally happy, gains weight reasonably well, and sucks his finger much of the day. This is considered normal by many. We don't believe it is normal for the baby to suck his fingers much of the time.

3. The baby starts to wake up frequently in the night when he previously woke up infrequently or not at all. Or, surprisingly, perhaps, on the contrary, now sleeps long hours during the night, perhaps sucking his thumb or a pacifier.

4. So-called "nursing strikes", which we no longer believe are a real diagnosis. The "nursing strike" is due to the baby's sense that there is not much milk in the breast and therefore he loses interest in the breast and doesn't latch on. Interestingly the babies who refuse the breast in the day, often feed better at night, at a time when most mothers have more milk.

5. Late onset sore nipples, with the baby "biting" or pulling at the breast. As well, when flow of milk slows, babies tend to slip down on the nipple, causing the mother nipple pain. They also tend to pull away from the breast, not

necessarily letting go of the breast, another way the mother starts having nipple pain.

6. Candida/yeast/thrush does not explain the above symptoms though the mother is frequently told this is the problem. Babies are not generally bothered by thrush.

7. Decrease in bowel movements. This may be normal, but we are beginning to rethink this and believe that if breastfeeding is associated with any of the other symptoms listed here, infrequent bowel movements cannot be called "normal".

8. The baby may start waking up more at night. This results in the baby getting more milk because, as mentioned already, babies tend to feed better in the night, and, as a result, this may be one reason that the baby continues to gain weight well in spite of other symptoms.

9. On the other hand, the baby may start sleeping during the night when he wasn't before, again a reaction to a decreased milk supply.

10. The baby is "self-weaning". We do not believe a baby younger than 2 or 3 years of age will "self wean". If they lose interest in taking the breast, it usually means the mother's milk supply has decreased.

How do we know the baby is "finished" the first side?

Because the baby is no longer drinking, even with breast compression. This does not mean the mother must take the baby off the breast as soon as the baby doesn't drink at all for a minute or two (the mother may get another milk ejection reflex or letdown reflex). However, if it is obvious the baby is not drinking, we recommend the mother take the baby off the breast and offer the other side, *before* the baby is very sleepy or fast asleep. If the baby is pulling at the breast and compressions are not helping, the mother should take the baby off the breast and offer the other side. If the baby is awake and no longer hungry, he won't take the second side. If the baby wants more, the baby will take the second side. If the baby becomes too sleepy while on the first breast, though, he may not take the second side. How do you know the baby is drinking or not?

If the baby lets go of the breast on his own, does it mean that the baby has "finished" that side? Not necessarily. Babies often let go of the breast when the flow of milk slows temporarily, or sometimes when the mother gets a milk ejection reflex and the baby, surprised by the sudden rapid flow, pulls off. The mother can try him again on that side if he wants more, but if the baby is obviously not drinking even with compression, she should switch sides. *Before* he gets too sleepy because if the baby is fast asleep, he might not take the second side even though he would if he were more awake.

WHO TRANSFERS THE MILK?

Our video on www.ibconline.ca is of a baby born at 35 weeks gestation, now 5 weeks old. The mother is breastfeeding and supplementing with a bottle. The video shows that the widely held notion that breastfeeding "tires out the baby" is false. Babies respond to milk flow. In the video, when the milk flow slowed, the baby started to fall asleep and the video starts with the baby essentially asleep and not sucking. When the flow is increased by supplementation with a lactation aid at the breast, the baby wakes up, opens his eyes and sucks vigorously. The video illustrates two related realities:

Which realities?

1. That young babies respond to milk flow and tend to fall asleep when the flow slows (Watch older babies may pull away from the breast when the flow slows) and this other reality,

2. Babies don't "transfer" milk, *mothers* transfer milk. The baby, of course, does his part, which is to stimulate the breast so that the milk flows from the breast to the baby. This is why a good latch helps the baby get more milk. When the baby latches on poorly, the breast is not stimulated well, and milk does not flow well from the breast. But the baby doesn't "suck the milk out of the breast".

In a video on www.ibconline.ca, *the 2 or 3 day old baby was not receiving milk well from the breast. To increase the amount of milk he receives, the mother was shown how to latch the baby on with an asymmetric latch. An improved latch and breast compressions resulted in the baby receiving significant amounts of milk.* **Go to www.ibconline.ca to watch the video.**

The above becomes obvious, we think, when we imagine a baby waking up from a sleep and perhaps starting to cry. Many mothers would have a milk ejection reflex (letdown reflex) and the front of their blouse would become wet. So, who transfers milk? Obviously, it's the mother. It is necessary to emphasize that the baby does his part, letting the mother know he's hungry, but it's the mother who transfers the milk.

What are some of the implications?

1. Breastfeeding is *not* tiring for the baby. Babies respond to milk flow. If the flow of milk is slow, the young baby tends to fall asleep, as in the video. The older baby may pull away from the breast, or fuss at the breast. If we increase the flow of milk, the "tired" baby suddenly is wide awake and sucks vigorously.

2. Babies (full term as well as prematures, such as **babies with cardiac problems, premature babies**) *do not* use up more energy breastfeeding than they do bottle feeding. This seems to be almost universal thinking at cardiology units and neonatal intensive care units in pediatric hospitals around the world. As a result of such thinking, mothers are told that they cannot breastfeed their babies because the baby will tire out from the breastfeeding and we need to conserve his energy. This is thought to be true even of healthy, full term babies.

3. It is *not* easier for the baby to feed from a bottle than from the breast. Too often pediatricians, neonatologists, and pediatric cardiologists, tell mothers not to breastfeed because it takes too much work for the baby to breastfeed and it's better to bottle feed.

4. Babies do not need "strong" muscles in their cheeks to breastfeed. This is said to be one of the reasons that "near term" babies have difficulties breastfeeding. It is not true that "near term" babies necessarily have difficulties breastfeeding. Babies much more **immature than 36 or 35 weeks gestation** can latch on and breastfeed just fine. What changes for "the worse" when the baby is born at 36 or 37 weeks, for example?

5. Babies are *not* "lazy". They respond to milk flow. And it follows that normal babies do not have "weak sucks", unless they are affected by medication or some other cause of depression of the nervous system. If the flow of milk from

131

the breast is relatively steady and rapid, the baby will suck just right and not fall asleep if he is latched on well.

6. We teach a method we call "**breast compression**" to increase the transfer of milk from the mother to the baby. It works very well much of the time. The method helps the mother transfer more milk to the baby. If mothers use breast compression to increase of flow of milk to the baby, they understand that, of course, mothers transfer milk, not babies.

7. "The more the baby sucks, the more milk the mother will make". This is simply not true. The mother does not make more milk simply because the baby is sucking for a long time. A baby "nibbling" on the breast is not receiving milk and not stimulating more milk production.

We think about babies and pumps working in the same way, and thus, the baby should keep sucking milk out of the breast, like a pump. Except that it is the mother who transfers the milk, not the baby. And even pumps do not get milk indefinitely.

And the result of this mistaken idea? Mothers keep babies on the breast for long periods of time thinking this will increase their milk supply. But a "nibbling" baby: does not increase the milk supply because babies do not transfer milk.

And when mothers need to supplement, using a **lactation aid at the breast**, they often do not introduce the lactation aid *early* enough. Many will wait *much* too long, when the baby has stopped drinking and is sitting on the breast nibbling away, not receiving milk. Thus, the baby is on the breast for long periods of time, and the lactation aid is blamed not only for the length of the feedings, but also that the lactation aid results in the mother producing less milk. Which is a strange notion. If anything, using the lactation aid at the breast increases the milk supply.

Watch a video on www.ibcoline.ca showing a baby who is hardly getting milk from the breast. He is nibbling only. He could sit nibbling on the breast for hours and still the mother's milk supply will not increase.

132

8. And why would **breast compression** help? Mothers transfer milk, not babies. Because the baby isn't doing his part as well as he could, and so breast compression compensates for his not doing his part as well as he could. And the reason the baby is not doing his part as well as he could? The baby is not as well latched on as well as he could be. And why is the baby not latched on as well as he could be?

a. The way the baby is latched on. The way the mother puts the baby to the breast can make all the difference in the world.

b. Use of artificial nipples such as bottles and **nipple shields** and pacifiers.

c. The baby has a **tongue tie**. Recently we saw a baby of 3 days of age with a very tight tongue tie. Before the release of his tongue tie, the baby was receiving almost no milk from the breast. After the release of the tongue tie, the increase in the amount of milk the baby received from the breast was dramatic. It is obvious that the milk supply and flow of milk to the baby did not increase dramatically in the 15 minutes between the first feeding before the tongue tie was released and the second feeding after the tongue tie release. What changed was how the baby latched on and the mother's response to the stimulation by the "new" latch. For this reason, tongue ties should be released early, before the mother's milk supply reduces. How we wish we had filmed this baby.

d. **A decrease in the mother's milk production** itself, can also result in a poor latch. How? Because when milk supply and flow of milk to the baby decrease, the baby tends to slip down on the breast to the nipple. If the baby is latched on only on the nipple, the milk flow to the baby decreases even more. And the mother may start to have late onset sore nipples.

WHEN THE BABY DOES NOT YET LATCH ON

When a baby does not yet latch on, it can be very distressing for the mother, her partner, for the hospital staff, and for the rest of the family. A baby who does not latch on represents the third most common problem we see at our clinic, not far behind the baby not getting enough from the breast and the mother who has sore nipples.

Why would a baby be incapable of latching on to the breast?

This problem would seem completely contrary to assuring survival of the baby and a baby not latching on must have been a very uncommon problem before modern medicine.

Many babies do not latch on because of **the way women now give birth** in the 21st century.

1. **Overhydration of the mother with intravenous fluids** during labour, birth and after the birth resulting in swelling of the mother's areolas and nipples, may make it very difficult for the baby to latch on. And too often, when the baby does not latch on immediately, instead of the hospital staff letting the mother and baby have some time to get used to each other and to get the baby latched on, the baby is started on bottles and/or the mother is given a **nipple shield**. The idea that a nipple shield actually does something good is an illusion. In fact, a baby on a nipple shield is not latched on at all, and the **milk supply decreases sooner or later**.

2. **Suctioning the baby after birth**. The first experience of the baby after birth, if negative, may result in the baby refusing to latch on. Oral stimulation in the newborn baby is a very powerful experience. Suctioning is a brutal procedure and a very strong, negative one for the baby who may develop an aversion to something, anything, being put into his mouth. And the worst of it all, is that suctioning is rarely necessary. Once, not that long ago, it was done to every baby, as a routine.

3. **Medications given during labour and birth.** For example, medications given for pain. Despite what many anaesthetists say, it is simply not true that medication given through an epidural does not affect the baby. See these studies: *Birth* 2001;28(1):5–12, *Anesthesiology* 2005;103(6):1211–1217, *Eur J Clin Pharmacol* 2005;61(7):517–522, *Int Breastfeed J* 2006;1:24, *Midwifery* 2009;25(2):e31–e38, *Matern Child Health J* 2013;17(4):689–698, *Birth* 2015;42(4):319-328

4. If the baby is separated from the mother after birth instead of being allowed to be skin to skin with the mother for at least 2 hours after the birth, the baby is much less likely to latch on, especially if he receives artificial nipples. A baby should be allowed to **crawl to the breast** from the mother's chest, but this is rarely done in most hospitals in the world because it takes time, up to 50 minutes and more, but sometimes less. But in the long run, this time is well spent.

Here's an anecdote: *A friend of mine's husband fainted during the birth of her first baby. The staff gave her the baby to hold while they attended to the father who had hit his head and was out cold. My friend, looking anxiously at her husband, did not notice at first that the baby, all by herself, had latched on and was suckling.*

5. A baby who is swaddled or wrapped up after birth is less likely to latch on. The layers of clothing may prevent the baby from being able to latch or from finding an easy way to latch on to the breast. Layers of clothing may also make the baby sleepy instead of alert and search for the breast. In a very real sense, a baby swaddled or wrapped up is separated from his mother.

6. **Studies** have shown that the baby finds the breast by smell. Washing the nipples and areolas may **make it more difficult for the baby to find the breast** and latch on. As does wiping or washing babies' hands.

7. Babies who have experienced problems such as lack of oxygen during birth and shortly afterwards and had to be resuscitated, may have difficulty latching on to the breast. This could be due to damage to the nervous system

135

(temporary or long lasting) or to the manipulations involved during resuscitation. Such babies are often quickly separated from their mothers and taken to the neonatal intensive care unit.

8. Forcing the baby into the breast and trying to force the baby to stay there, is not going to work. The baby will either go limp or fight the breast, pushing away from the breast. Some babies may go limp one time and cry and push away from the breast another. Too often the "helper" will keep trying to force the baby into the breast, which only makes things worse.

Other reasons a baby may not latch on:

1. **Tongue tie** alone, unless very severe, probably does not prevent a baby from latching on, but combine a tongue tie with a mother's breasts that are swollen from intravenous fluids, the baby all swaddled and thus separated from his mother, and early introduction of bottles because the baby is not latching on and we have a problem. Breastfeeding problems, including a baby who will not latch on, are usually due to several issues acting together. The tongue tie is only one of a combination of things that result in the baby not latching on.

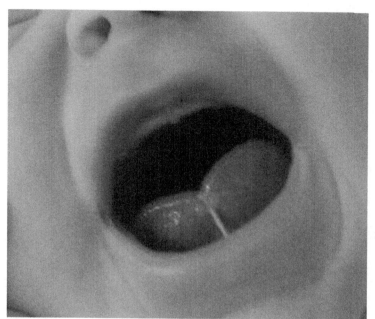

This baby's tongue tie is quite obvious, though the mother was told by the hospital staff, that he didn't have a tongue tie. Tongue ties may make latching on more difficult for the baby. Tongue ties also often cause the mother sore nipples.

2. Babies with cleft palates have difficulty latching on. But **some babies do manage it**. Unfortunately, some cleft palate programmes assume the baby will not latch on and will simply tell the mother *not even to try* breastfeeding. Obviously, if the baby is never even tried on the breast, he won't latch on. In some cleft palate programmes babies are immediately fitted with an obturator to close the gap and babies with these obturators apparently do latch on, at least many of them do.

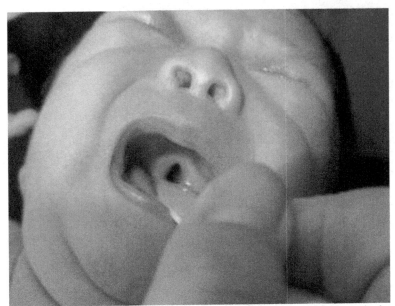

This is a typical cleft of the soft palate. It was missed in hospital because too often physical examination of the newborn is perfunctory. In the case of a cleft of the soft palate, often the baby allows the breast into his mouth (but doesn't really latch on) and makes a typical clucking sound when sucking.

3. Some mothers have very large nipples or infolded nipples (sometimes called inverted nipples). Infolded nipples in themselves should not make breastfeeding impossible.

In fact, very large or very long nipples are probably more of a problem than infolded nipples. But taking the time for the baby to learn how to latch on to those breasts with very large nipples will eventually pay off. Feed the baby, by cup, by spoon. The **lactation aid at the breast** will often work even if the nipples are very large. The baby gets used to getting milk from the breast and eventually the baby will "get it" and latch on. Patience is a virtue in these situations. Rushing in with bottles or a **nipple shield** is not a virtue.

4. Babies with neurological or some other (facial/oral) abnormalities may have difficulties latching on.

If the baby is not latching on, what do we do?

1. Have patience, don't panic straight away after birth and rush in with "solutions" such bottles and **nipple shield**.

2. Skin to skin contact, as much as possible, and the baby may find the breast and latch on, sometimes without any help at all. A nurse or other qualified health professional should be with the mother and baby, as the mother and the baby both may some residual effects from the medication the mother has received.

3. If the baby has not latched on within a few hours, the mother should get help to express her milk and feed the baby with a spoon or open cup. Hand expression often works better than a pump before the milk increases on day 3 or 4. And often even if the milk has increased.

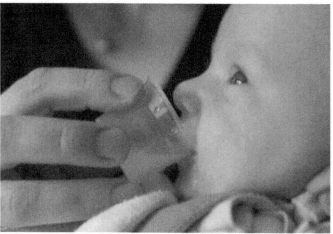

This baby is being cup fed with his mother's expressed colostrum. Why is a bottle better? It's not.

Watch a video (www.ibconline.ca) in which a 4 month old baby is being fed with an open cup so as to avoid using a bottle. Cup feeding is possible even if the baby is a day old or and even premature. And even in this case where the baby has a significant tongue tie.

4. The mother should get qualified, skilled help to **get the baby to latch on well**.

5. Use of **breast compression** to increase the flow of milk from the breast which will encourage the baby to latch on and stay on.

6. Hospital staff should create a relaxed atmosphere around all babies but particularly around those who do not latch on immediately. Panic by the staff is not going to help. If the staff panics, so will the mother. Many babies will latch on when the milk supply increases on day 3 or 4.

7. After day 3 or 4 when the mother's milk supply has increased and the baby is still not latching on, **finger feeding** is a technique that frequently works to prepare the baby to take the breast. The video below shows how finger feeding works to latch the baby on. Note that the finger feeding need be done only a very short time before trying the baby on the breast. Finger feeding wakes up a sleepy baby and also calms down a fussy baby.

Watch a video on www.ibconline.ca which shows how finger feeding is a useful technique to help a baby who is reluctant to latch on to latch on. Finger feeding calms an upset baby and wakes up a sleepy baby. Once the baby is sucking well, move the baby over to the breast. Do not try to force the baby into the breast and hold him there so that he will take the breast. Trying to force the baby into the breast when he resists staying there, only makes things worse. As seen in the video (www.ibconline.ca), it took a couple of tries to get the baby to latch on. Letting the baby come off the breast if he has not latched on works better than trying to keep the baby pushed into the breast, which usually does not work at all, but usually makes things worse. This baby was born several weeks prematurely, is now 2 months old in the video and has never before in his life latched on.

8. Using the **lactation aid at the breast** after finger feeding may be a good way to help the baby stay on the breast. The use of a lactation aid to keep the baby on the breast is seen in our videos on www.ibconline.ca.

9. Some babies are willing to experiment with latching on if they were first fed a little bit of milk via finger feeding or cup feeding. A ravenous baby may not be patient enough to take the breast but decreasing his hunger somewhat by feeding by open cup or finger feeding may result in his latching on.

10. Trying to latch the baby on right after the baby wakes up or just as the baby is falling asleep sometimes works very well. See point 9.

11. Babies who are crying and screaming are difficult to latch on. Showing the mother how to calm the baby can help the baby to latch on.

12. Making sure the mother expresses her milk and builds up a very good milk supply. An abundant milk supply is a major determinant of whether the baby will eventually latch on. More milk means faster flow, faster flow means the baby is more likely to latch on. But when mothers don't have a lot of milk, the baby will often still latch on when we use the methods mentioned above. And if the baby starts to latch on regularly, the mother's milk will increase, and, more importantly, the flow of milk from mother to baby will increase.

Patience, yes, is a virtue. Even at the beginning of the 19th century, before epidurals, before intravenous infusions, babies did not always latch on immediately. What does it tell us? Not to put too fine a point on it, that babies do not always latch on immediately, but patience, a little patience, and often the baby will do it. Read this small part of Goethe's play, Faust, and you will give good advice and, at wisdom's copious breasts, you too will know how to do the right thing for a baby who is not latching on.

The child, offered the mother's breast,
Will not in the beginning grab it;
But soon it clings to it with zest.
And thus at wisdom's copious breasts
You'll drink each day with greater zest.

So nimmt ein Kind der Mutter Brust
Nicht gleich im Anfang willig an,
Doch bald ernährt es sich mit Lust.

So wird's Euch an der Weisheit Brüsten
Mit jedem Tage mehr gelüsten.

—Goethe. Faust. Mephistopheles speaking to the student

And domperidone?

Even if the mother is able to express all the milk the baby needs, we will often use domperidone to increase the mother's milk supply. Why? Because more milk means faster flow of milk from the breast and faster flow means the baby is more likely to latch on. Go back to the **video of the baby latched on after finger feeding**. You will notice that the baby is latched on with a lactation aid at the breast. The baby gets more flow of milk and thus latches on and stays on the breast, though it takes a couple of tries.

WHAT ABOUT NIPPLE SHIELDS?

The use of nipple shields has become almost epidemic in North America and Europe. Nipple shields are seen as the answer to virtually *all* breastfeeding problems, from babies not latching on, to nipple soreness, to *routine* use for premature babies. Even the perception of a mother's nipples being "flat" often results in the recommendation of a nipple shield sometimes without even an attempt to latch the baby at the breast. We have heard stories from mothers attending our clinic that they were given a nipple shield immediately after the birth of the baby, *before* they had even tried to put the baby to the breast, simply based on the *appearance* of the nipples. And were the mothers able to get the baby to take the breast without the nipple shield? Yes, with our help.

This "epidemic" has occurred without any evidence that nipple shields are safe to use and actually do what they are supposed to do. A quote from a **review of the literature** on nipple shields says it all: "Introducing nipple shields in the first postpartum week may seem like an easy fix for a frustrated family, but such intervention may preclude a thorough evaluation of the mother–infant dyad to determine **why breastfeeding has been problematic** and may cause more problems such as **lack of effective milk transfer, sore nipples, and loss of milk supply.** The pervasive use of nipple shields as an intervention in the very early course of breastfeeding can relay a false message of breastfeeding success and safety to mothers. Widespread retail access to nipple shields might also signal to mothers that nipple shield use is a norm that warrants little concern." **In clinical medicine, it is generally accepted that one must prove the *safety* and *usefulness* of an intervention** before one can generally recommend it. Nipple shield use has never been proved safe or effective. Nipple shields have never passed this requirement.

The nipple shield is a recommendation without regard to the long term, not only when recommended in the first few days but even in the mother whose baby has started to refuse the breast due to **late onset decreased milk supply** when there are much more rational and effective treatments. But it is particularly pernicious when used to get the baby to take the breast when so many babies who do not latch on during the first few days would easily latch on when the milk supply and milk flow increase on day 3 or 4, especially if the mother is helped by someone skilled at helping with **latching on**. The questions that are not asked are: "How will a mother whose baby is on a nipple shield continue breastfeeding long term?", "How will the mother in such a case be able to stop using the nipple shield?", "What will the effect of the nipple shield be on her milk supply both in the short and **longer term**?", "What are other side effects of the use of nipple shields?". And "What happens to these mothers and babies when they forget the nipple shield on leaving home with the baby who otherwise does not take the breast?"

Is there are better way?

The most important question is whether something else could have been done instead of introducing a nipple shield. We are convinced, based on more than 45 years of combined experience helping mothers with breastfeeding that **there is nothing that can be done with a nipple shield than cannot be done better without one**. If a baby can latch on to a nipple shield, the baby should be able to latch on to the breast.

The basic problem is that the more nipple shields are used, the less experience people have searching for and applying alternative solutions, including learning how to **help a mother help her baby latch on**. The nipple shield solution seems to be an attractive one because it *appears* to work quickly, indeed, immediately, in most cases. People do love quick solutions.

Unfortunately, patience, skill and experience are necessary to solve some breastfeeding problems; both the mother and the person wanting to help her need to be patient. There is nothing terrible about waiting a few days to get a baby to **latch on**, if, in the meantime, the mother is given the tools to feed her baby during this time. Even newborn babies can drink from an open cup and/or be fed from a small spoon.

We would also suggest that a large part of a postpartum nurse's, lactation consultant's work is to counsel the mother and part of this is to counsel patience and provide the kind of temporary solution that leads to *successful breastfeeding long term*. Let us propose that for each problem for which a nipple shield is used, there is a *real* solution which takes into account the long term perspective.

So, what are the problems with the use of nipple shields?

1. Let us be frank: A baby on a nipple shield is not latched on, not at all; it is an illusion to believe he is. Breastfeeding with a nipple shield is not the same as breastfeeding directly. No matter how thin the nipple shield, it's still not the breast. The question is: if feeding through a nipple shield is "just like breastfeeding", then why will a baby seemingly "take the breast" with a nipple shield and not take the breast directly? Instead of the baby latching on to the naked breast, the soft, supple, pliable breast, latching on to the breast being an active process, the nipple shield, which is not soft, supple, or pliable, is essentially pushed into the baby's mouth. The "nipple" of the nipple shield has a much harder texture than the mother's nipple and is wider and longer. The nipple shield makes the breast into a bottle, essentially. With a nipple shield in his mouth, the baby uses his tongue and cheek muscles just as he does on a bottle or a pacifier and not the way he would when breastfeeding. When a baby is on a nipple shield, in order to get milk, the baby needs to suck hard to get milk out of the breast. This is not **what a baby does on the breast**. When a baby feeds directly from the breast, he is using a whole different process. He **stimulates the breast to release the milk which then flows to the baby**. And this is obvious because it is so difficult in most cases to get a baby who is hooked on a nipple shield to then take the breast directly. If they were the same as so many suggest, then why is that so?

2. Some people believe that nipple shields are a tool for teaching a baby how to breastfeed. This is the reason they are used so frequently in the premature baby. But as stated above, this is pure fantasy. A nipple shield teaches a premature baby how to suck from a nipple shield, but not how to breastfeed.

3. A baby on a nipple shield is actually not latched on. A baby on a nipple shield will never do what he is supposed to do on the breast. And delatching a baby from a nipple shield is extremely easy to do, not as it would be if he were directly latched on well to the naked breast.

145

4. One of the most common reasons for **milk supply to decrease with time** is that the baby's latch is not as good as it could be. For example, when the baby has a **tongue tie**. Since a baby on a nipple shield is not latched on at all, with time, the milk supply may, and often does, decrease significantly. The reason this is controversial is that in a small number of cases, when a mother begins with an abundant milk supply, she and the baby may manage for several months; however, if the milk supply decreases enough, the baby will start to refuse to take the nipple-shielded breast and/or become very unhappy even on the nipple shield, never mind the breast, with the result that the mother introduces bottle supplements. This often occurs within weeks of birth. As an aside, if the mother's milk supply had been so abundant, it should have been easy to get the baby to latch on in the first week of life. In fact, many mothers are able to get the baby to take the breast directly after weeks of the baby drinking through a nipple shield, precisely because the mother started off with an abundant milk supply. Even then, we would suggest that the milk supply had decreased, but luckily, was still adequate for the baby to receive milk well from the breast.

5. When the flow of milk is diminished due to a poor latch, including due to nipple shield use, the mother may begin to have problems with **recurrent blocked ducts, mastitis and even breast abscess**. Blocked ducts/mastitis occur at first when the mother has a fairly generous milk supply, but the baby's latch is not good, and the breast does not drain well. The exact situation of a baby sucking on a nipple shield.

6. Even though nipple shields are supposed to treat sore nipples, in fact, some mothers actually develop nipple pain while on nipple shields. And for some, the pain is in fact *worse* while she is using the nipple shield.

7. To reiterate, once the baby is habituated to the nipple shield, it is difficult for that baby to start to take the breast directly. Mothers intrinsically understand that using a nipple shield is **not really what they wanted**, but what we may have done is taken true breastfeeding, that is, *on the breast*, away from them. Those of us working with mothers and babies on a nipple shield find it is much more difficult to get the baby breastfeeding directly from the breast than if the baby were on a bottle, which is not to say that the bottle is a solution either.

146

Young babies who are not latching on can be fed by spoon or open cup. The older the baby on a nipple shield is, the more difficult it is to get rid of the nipple shield.

8. A very big problem associated with the use of nipple shields is that the mother believes that the nipple shield has corrected her problems and she may see no need to do anything further, until it's too late. Typically, a mother coming to us for help, has had a **decrease in her milk supply** because of the nipple shield and has found that her baby fusses at the nipple-shielded breast, is not satisfied and not getting as much milk as before. And the longer this goes on, the more difficult it is to get the baby to the breast. So, nipple shield + decrease in milk supply due to nipple shield = greater and greater difficulty in latching the baby on. Often, the mother finds she is not only using a nipple shield but also giving the baby bottles to her fussy baby.

Even if some believe that nipple shields do treat certain breastfeeding problems, the risks associated with the use of nipple shields (see above), should give us pause. Any medical treatment or device that causes so many problems, would not be approved for use by any regulatory agency. And the nipple shield has not been approved.

Preventing the "need" for nipple shields

The causes of early breastfeeding problems include, **modern birthing practices, not allowing the baby to crawl** to the breast immediately after birth, no skin to skin contact between mother and baby, separation of mother and baby often for unnecessary reasons, early introduction of artificial nipples, feeding by the clock, and the use of % **weight loss** to determine the adequacy of breastfeeding.

Babies often will have difficulty latching on after a birth because of the large **amounts of intravenous fluids** given to the mother during labour, birth and after. Intravenous fluids during labour and birth go to the baby as well as to the mother and so result in the baby being "overhydrated" at birth and thus the **baby loses more weight**, approaches **the dreaded 10% weight loss** (for which, incidentally, there is no scientific basis) and panic begins to overtake the staff in hospital, panic which is transmitted to the parents.

In addition, the mother's nipples are often oedematous due to her being overhydrated and thus the baby has difficulty latching on. The answer to dealing with these issues is to help the mother get the baby well latched on. This may require **"reverse pressure softening"** of the breast. And it also requires knowing **how to know a baby is getting milk from the breast, or not getting milk from the breast**. The answer is not a nipple shield.

Nipple "shape" is a frequent excuse for giving the mother a nipple shield. Intravenous fluids are one cause of "flat nipples". Amazingly the nipples are no longer flat after the mother has had a diuresis (increased urine output), which starts immediately after the intravenous infusion has stopped, but may not be complete for a week and perhaps longer. This is too late if she has started a nipple shield, because she is usually now home, and believing, perhaps, that her problem has been solved. One of our patients had a nipple shield slapped on her breast while she was still on the delivery table, before she even tried to put the baby to the breast the first time. Interestingly, with a little help at our clinic, the baby latched on, though not without considerable difficulty. But latch on he did, and went on to breastfeed exclusively, not nipple shield feed. No shape of nipple – "flat", "inverted", "large" – should make it *impossible* for a baby to latch on and to be a reason for using a nipple shield.

The most common reasons for mothers being advised to use a nipple shield are the following: 1. The baby is not latching on. 2. The mother has sore nipples and 3. The baby is premature.

Dealing with a non-latching baby without a nipple shield

Some babies just do not latch on from the very beginning, many for reasons that are not obvious. It seems that people always knew this. At the beginning of the 19th century, Goethe remarked on this in his drama *Faust* where Mephistopheles says to the student:

So nimmt ein Kind der Mutter Brust
Nicht gleich im Anfang willig an,
Doch bald ernährt es sich mit Lust.

So wird's Euch an der Weisheit Brüsten
Mit jedem Tage mehr gelüsten.

Here is what I've been told is not the best of all translations of Goethe:

The child, offered the mother's breast,
Will not in the beginning grab it;
But soon it clings to it with zest.
And thus at wisdom's copious breasts
You'll drink each day with greater zest.

Current hospital practices are geared to instant solutions, but this "gotta fix it now, this very minute, approach" needs to change and an atmosphere should be created in which mothers and babies are not rushed or forced to get the baby to the breast as soon as possible, immediately.

It is frequent, indeed, almost routine, that many mothers will have an **intravenous during labour,** birth and after and this may result in oedema of the nipples and areolas. This oedema will regress, which is important to appreciate and if appreciated, will help us develop the patience that is necessary to avoid jumping in with a nipple shield. It is also frequent that mothers will receive epidural and/or spinal analgesia. The evidence is strong that the **drugs used do indeed affect the baby** and result in babies being "confused" or too sleepy. Again, patience is important. So what to do?

• The breast crawl: the baby is skin to skin with the mother immediately after birth and allowed to crawl to the breast and latch on without help, is of supreme importance. It takes precedence over weighing the baby, washing the baby and so many other routine practices that interfere with the breast crawl and latching on of the baby. The breast crawl may take an hour or more and obviously clashes with the current hospital ambiance and practices.

• Even after the initial breast crawl, mothers and babies should be skin to skin as much as possible.

• Every baby should be checked at birth for **tongue tie even if the breastfeeding seems to be going well.** Checking for tongue tie should be as routine as checking the baby's breathing or listening to his heart. However, the majority of health professionals do not know how to decide if a baby has a tongue tie or not, very frequently passing off a very obvious tongue tie as "normal" or "of no significance".

• As soon as there is a concern that the baby is not latching on or does not actually drink from the breast, the mother's milk should be expressed and fed to the baby by spoon or open cup and not by bottle. This is not the time to introduce a nipple shield! In our opinion, there is never a time to introduce a nipple shield.

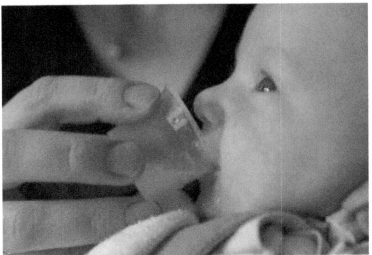

This baby is being fed expressed breastmilk by cup, which is better than a bottle and a useful approach to avoid a nipple shield.

• Hospital staff, including midwives, nursing staff, physicians and lactation consultants need to know how to help a reluctant baby latch on when he is showing early signs of being ready to feed. There is a real technique to **helping babies latch on well** and those who use nipple shields from their earliest training never learn this technique.

• The mother should be reassured that her baby will eventually latch on and she should start a routine of hand expression of her milk, cup and/or spoon feeding and she should be taught the **"technique" of latching on her baby**.

• Followup of any baby not latching on should be within a day or two of discharge from hospital by someone who is experienced in helping reluctant babies latch on. Once the milk increases ("comes in"), it is sometimes much easier to help the baby to latch on.

Dealing with sore nipples without a nipple shield

Sore nipples are almost always due to a baby's **less than adequate latch**. No matter what the latch looks like from the outside, if the mother has pain, something is wrong with how the baby is latching on to the breast.

An anecdote. About 2 years ago, I was called to see the new grandchild of a good friend of mine. The baby was 36 hours old when I arrived. The mother was starting to have sore nipples and the baby was never satisfied after a feeding and cried constantly. It took me 1 minute to fix the problem by helping the mother **latch the baby on** differently from what she was doing. I also taught her **breast compression** and for the first time the baby fed well and was calm. I should say that in many cases, this is very possible and much easier to deal with than if the baby had been 3 weeks old and on a nipple shield.

So, the key to preventing problems such as sore nipples is to make sure the baby has **a good latch** and that the baby is drinking well from the breast. This means that soon after the baby is born, on the first day, someone should observe a feeding and if the mother complains of pain, something needs to be done, and that something is not "try a nipple shield". If examination of the baby reveals a tongue tie, release of the tongue tie should not be deferred. Sore nipples should not be considered "normal".

Other measures, such as the use of ointments on the nipple can be used as *stop gaps*. A nipple shield is neither a stop gap nor the answer.

Dealing with premature babies

Nipple shields are not a method of teaching premature or any other babies "how to suck". Babies learn to breastfeed *by breastfeeding* and getting milk from the breast.

Based on work particularly from Scandinavia but also in other sites including Columbia, babies can and should be going to the breast, without a nipple shield it must be said, **by 27 or so weeks gestation**. The North American approach of "no breastfeeding until 34 weeks gestation" has been shown to be detrimental to premature babies learning to breastfeed. The idea that they need to learn to bottle feed before they can start breastfeeding is bizarre to say the least and based on the false notion that **breastfeeding is tiring, or "hard work"**.

So, what about mothers who say that the nipple shield saved their breastfeeding?

We will repeat it: **there is nothing that can be done with a nipple shield that cannot be done *better* without one**. Measures can be taken to help mothers with breastfeeding problems which would have prevented the "need" for the nipple shield in the first place. The reason we hear stories that "the nipple shield saved my breastfeeding" is the same as those stories that "The doctor said that if I didn't take this antibiotic for my cold, I could have become much sicker" or "a couple of bottles of formula in the first days saved my breastfeeding". A couple of bottles of formula in the first days saved my breastfeeding may be true, but there was still a better way and one that does not include the risks of formula feeding. For each mother who believes that the nipple shield saved her breastfeeding, there are countless mothers whose breastfeeding was marked by decreasing milk supply, breast refusal, painful nipples and premature weaning. The means, the methods we use to help mothers with breastfeeding problems are important and should be those means that allow the mother and baby to develop the skills that lead to a happy and long term breastfeeding relationship.

IS MY BABY GETTING ENOUGH MILK? (PART 1)

Why would a breastfeeding baby not be getting enough breastmilk? It is true that some mothers really cannot produce all the milk the babies need. In some cases, because the mother has hormonal issues as in polycystic ovarian syndrome, or because the mother has had **breast reduction surgery** or other surgery where the incision has been made around the areola. However, most frequently, the most important reason is that **the baby is not latched on as well as he could be**. If the baby is not latched on well, the baby does not stimulate the breast as well as he could and thus the milk does not flow well from the mother to the baby (note that **mothers transfer milk, not babies**).

And why would a baby not be latched on as well as he could be?

Because of:

1. How the baby is positioned and latched on. **Mothers are frequently told that "the baby's latch is perfect". It is easy to say so, but in our experience, the vast majority of babies we see at our clinic are *not* latching on as well as they could be. A less than ideal latch does not necessarily mean a latch that is "not good enough". When mothers start off with a very good milk supply, babies may get enough milk, but it is also possible that with time, the milk supply will decrease.

2. **The use of artificial nipples such as bottles, pacifiers and** nipple shields. It is unfortunate that the first thing many mothers are advised to do when there are problems with breastfeeding is to give the baby formula, usually with a bottle, which serves to increase the weight, but does not address the real issue and very often makes the breastfeeding go downhill. When it is determined that the baby truly needs supplementation, **a lactation aid at the breast is a far better way to supplement a baby** (not an SNS), but the mother needs to be shown how to use it so that it works well. The baby's **latch** needs to be as good as possible and the tube of the lactation aid needs to be well placed. One without the other makes the use of the lactation aid at the breast difficult.

3. **The baby has a** tongue tie. Some tongue ties are obvious, but many tongue ties are more subtle and require an evaluation that goes further than just looking. Evaluation requires feeling under the baby's tongue as well, assessing the *upward mobility of the tongue* and, of course, knowing what to feel for. Unfortunately, few health professionals, including many lactation consultants, know how to evaluate whether or not the baby has a tongue tie. As well, not all health professionals know how to release a tongue tie properly. Too often, partial release may not really help much. It should also be noted that a tongue tie interferes with the baby's latching on and so makes the use of the lactation aid more difficult as a result.

4. **Decreased milk supply, (which does not mean "not enough milk" but rather a *decrease* in milk supply relative to what the baby was used to) can lead to even more decrease in the milk supply**. Late onset decreased milk supply is not uncommon (We see one or two mothers and babies every day at our clinic with late onset decreased milk supply). When the milk flow slows, the baby tends to slip down on the nipple and the latch becomes even worse, so that *decreased milk supply itself* can lead to even more of a decrease in milk flow. As this happens, in response to the slow flow of milk, most babies will stay on the breast drinking for shorter and shorter periods of time which contributes to the milk supply decreasing even further. And this may also result in the mother developing a new onset of sore nipples. *Watch our videos on www.ibconline.ca which showing babies drinking at the breast or not.*

The first few days

It is commonly believed that there is not enough milk for the baby in the first few days. This is bizarre thinking, imagining that babies can get dehydrated and even die because there is not enough milk. But the problem is not that there is not enough milk; in fact, there is, *almost always*, enough. Breastmilk has been produced in the breasts since about 16 weeks of pregnancy. The usual problem is that the baby *does not receive the milk that is available* to him.

And why does a baby not receive the milk that is available to him? Basically, because the baby is not latched on well. **How a baby latches on** determines how well he gets milk from the breast and this is particularly important when there are not large volumes of milk as in the first 3 or 4 days. The problem is that the importance of how a baby latches on is ignored in general unless the mother has **sore nipples,** and even when mothers have sore nipples the mother is often told the latch is just fine. (Secret: if the mother has **nipple pain** while breastfeeding, the latch is *not* good no matter who says otherwise and how it looks from the outside). And even if the health professional knows that the latch is important, few really know how to help the baby latch on well. Unfortunately, it is not a routine part of postpartum care in most hospitals to observe the baby at the breast and to help the mother with the latching on should it be necessary.

And most hospital staff are not aware how difficult it can be for a baby to latch on well when the mother's nipples and areolas are swollen from the **intravenous fluids given to the mother during labour and birth.** Mothers are often told that they have "flat nipples" and thus breastfeeding will never work for them. Unfortunately, far too often, the "treatment" of "flat nipples" is a **nipple shield.** When we see such mothers in the breastfeeding clinic, they do not have "flat nipples", they have normal nipples, as do the vast majority of mothers. The nipples had *looked* flat because of swelling due to the intravenous fluids. Telling the mother her nipples are "flat" is wrong and **undermines her confidence to breastfeeding and too often leads to the use of nipple shields.**

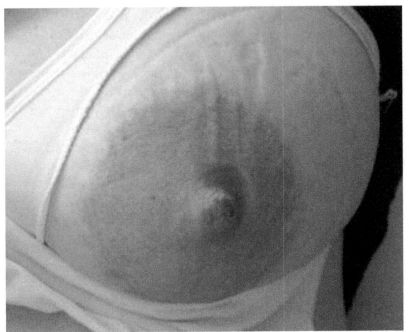

This mother has swelling of the breast, the nipple and the areola, due to retention of fluid. This makes it difficult for the baby to latch on. The result? The baby does not get milk well and the mother's nipples are sore.

Furthermore, *because* the mother and baby have been overloaded with fluid, *because* the baby does not latch on well, *because* of these factors and others, babies are supplemented, very often *without* any attempt to help the baby get milk from the breast by improving the **latching on**, *without* showing the mother **breast compression** to help the baby get more milk. As a result, the mother is convinced, by the "information" from the nurse, physician and lactation consultant, that she does not have enough milk. Too often this becomes a self-fulfilling prophecy.

The mother then continues the supplements, usually by bottle, which continues to undermine the baby's latch, which results in the baby getting less milk and as a result, more bottles and more formula. And often, that is the end of breastfeeding, sooner or later, too often sooner rather than later.

Watch a video on www.ibconline.ca which shows a baby who is 24 hours old and is drinking lots of milk from the breast. How do we know? Because of the pause in the chin as he opens his mouth wide to the maximum. The longer the pause, the more milk the baby received.

After the first few days

Are there truly women who cannot produce enough milk? Of course, this has always been and likely always will be. Probably, in tribal societies, when a baby was obviously not thriving, the baby would be shared around and fed by other nursing mothers as well as the mother herself. Just as with any other part of the human body, things can go wrong through no fault of the person affected.

Once humans started domesticating cattle, goats and sheep, babies were still shared around but they might also have received cow, sheep, mule, camel or mare milk. And many would have died from infection or quite possibly electrolyte imbalances if they were fed *only* animal milk. But even many of these babies usually did survive, because they received unpasteurized milk, sometimes directly from the animal. The milk would have contained immune factors, though immune factors appropriate for the animal.

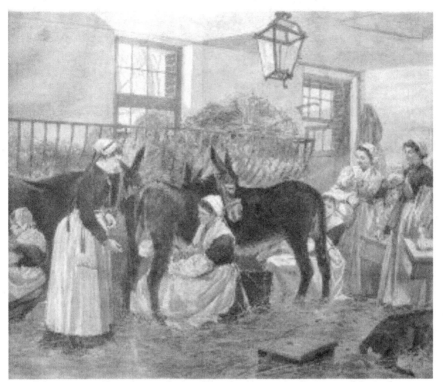

In 19th century France, orphans for whom a wet nurse could not be found, were sometimes fed directly at the teat of a domesticated animal, in this case, a donkey.

But, until mothers and babies get the help they need to establish and continue breastfeeding, there will always be far more mothers who *incorrectly* believe they are incapable of breastfeeding exclusively.

Why might a baby not get all the breastmilk that is available?

1. **Restricting time on the breast.** Mothers are still, *still* being told that the baby should be feeding a limited amount of time on the breast (say, 10 or 15 minutes on each breast) which might result in the baby not getting enough milk from the breast. There are some health professionals who *still* seem to believe that 10 minutes on the breast is enough because the baby gets 90% of the milk in that time. We really have no idea where this notion arose (that the baby gets 90% of the milk in the first 10 minutes of suckling).

2. **Feeding on schedule.** Many health professionals tell mothers that the baby should be offered the breast only every 3 hours or even 4 hours. Feeding only every three or four hours can cause the baby not to get enough milk and eventually for the mother's milk production to decrease. Most young babies are showing signs of hunger well before 3 or 4 hours. If the mother believes the "rule", the baby may be offered a pacifier instead of the breast. Pacifiers may decrease the milk supply because the baby is not on the breast. As a result, the pacifier is used more and more, because the baby is frequently fussy, wanting more milk, not a pacifier. Babies should be breastfed whenever they show signs of readiness to feed and they show readiness to feed *well before* they begin to cry.

3. **The use of pacifiers** can result both in a decrease in milk production and their use can also be a consequence of a decrease in milk production when the mother uses a pacifier to calm a baby who would actually need to go to the breast instead. The baby seems hungry well before he "is supposed to", so a pacifier is offered. The baby sucks on a pacifier instead of breastfeeding, and so milk production decreases, and the baby "needs" the pacifier even more. Eventually, the mother is advised by the baby's physician that the baby is not gaining enough, and she should supplement the baby with bottles of formula. We see a lot of *recent onset pacifier use* in babies whose mothers have had **late onset decreased milk supply.**

4. Feeding only one breast per feeding. The idea, apparently, is that the baby would get high fat milk. However, if the baby is not getting milk from the breast, he is not getting high fat milk. **A baby is not necessary getting milk simply because he is making sucking motions on the breast.**

Most mothers whose babies are not getting enough milk from the breast, are not getting enough because of a cascade of events that include birth interventions, **including use of** medications in the epidurals, **separation of mother and baby after birth, early and unnecessary use of artificial nipples, postpartum practices and bad breastfeeding advice. Thus, most causes of "insufficient milk supply" are preventable and potentially reversible if skilled help is begun early.**

159

Other causes of "insufficient milk supply"

1. **Women who have had** breast reduction surgery, which is most often done with an incision around the areola, *usually* do not produce enough milk. Recently, we have seen one mother who had breast reduction with liposuction, but we are unsure how this procedure affects breastmilk production. Furthermore, we have seen mothers in our clinic who have had breast reduction with the usual surgery and who *did* produce all the milk the baby needed. We even have seen one mother who had breast reduction who breastfed *twins* exclusively to 6 months of age. It should be mentioned that *any* breast surgery done with an incision made around the areola, will decrease the mother's capacity to make milk. The more complete the incision (breast reduction usually involves an incision completely around the areola), the greater the negative effect on milk production.

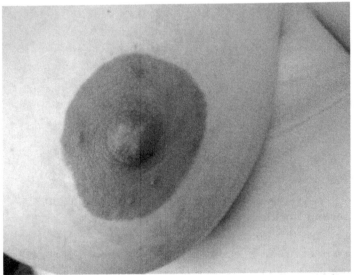

This mother has had breast reduction surgery. As a result, it has been difficult for her to produce enough milk for her baby.

2. It should be mentioned also that simply looking at a woman's breast is not a good way to determine whether she can produce enough milk or not.

160

Sometimes breasts are described as having "insufficient glandular tissue" (IGT). We do not like this term because it is essentially saying to the mother that she will never produce enough milk, and this is not true. This diagnosis is not helpful because it may cause the mother to feel insecure and it does not change how we would help the mother with breastfeeding.

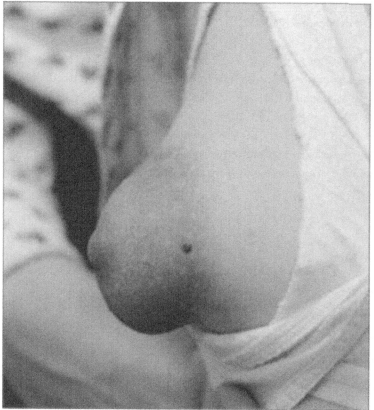

A mother with the typical signs of "insufficient glandular tissue". Her other breast also showed signs of "insufficient glandular tissue" but the baby gained well exclusively breastfeeding. Be careful making this diagnosis.

3. Women who **induce lactation to feed an adopted baby or a baby born with a surrogate** often do not produce all the milk the baby needs. But some do. And

mothers who wish to **relactate**, often do not produce all the milk the baby needs. But some do.

4. And there are some mothers who do not produce enough milk for reasons that are uncommon or unknown. Some of these uncommon causes include women who have had surgical removal of or damage to their pituitary gland or bilateral mastectomies.

Can these mothers breastfeed?

Of course, but they may not be able to breastfeed exclusively. **Part 2 of this chapter will discuss a practical approach to helping mothers breastfeed their babies as exclusively as possible.** Please understand, however, that breastfeeding is much more than just making milk for the baby. There is much more to breastfeeding than breastmilk. Breastfeeding is not just bottle feeding with a softer bottle. It is a close, **intimate physical and emotional relationship** between two people who are generally in love with each other.

IS MY BABY GETTING ENOUGH MILK? (PART 2)

Our approach to increasing the baby's intake of breastmilk when the baby is not getting as much as the mother and we would like is based on four principles:

1. When breastfeeding goes well, it is *easy* and *pleasant* for the mother and the baby. When breastfeeding is not going well, it should be as easy and as pleasant for the mother and baby as is possible given the circumstances.

2. First and foremost, we attempt to correct the difficulties without jumping to supplementation and bottles.

3. Breastfeeding is much more than breastmilk. Breastfeeding is a close, physical and emotional relationship between two people who are usually in love with each other.

4. It is possible to breastfeed even if the baby needs to be supplemented.

Thus, when breastfeeding is not going well, what does this mean in terms of our approach?

1. This means that as long as the baby is latching on reasonably well on the breast and receiving milk, that we do not encourage the mother to express or pump her milk as a way to increase milk supply. Pumping and hand expression are work, time consuming work, and we believe that when a mother feels obliged to pump or express her milk, she is likely to stop breastfeeding much earlier than if she does not pump or express her milk. Or she is much more likely to go to exclusive pumping and bottle feeding.

There is evidence that what a mother can express, or pump is not the same as what the baby receives from the breast. As well, we hear from many mothers, whose babies *are* gaining well breastfeeding exclusively, cannot express or pump much milk at all. A baby who is well latched on can get much more than what a mother might be able to pump. A baby poorly latched on will get less milk. Thus, in case the mother is told to pump in order to increase her milk supply and she gets very little milk, she might become discouraged and think that her baby also gets very little from the breast and give up breastfeeding altogether.

On the other hand, if the mother is able to express all the milk the baby needs, she should have been able to feed the baby exclusively at the breast and therefore the approach should be not to just say, "That's fine, wonderful", but help her so that the baby can get the milk from the breast.

Breast compression is like pumping but instead of pumping into a container, the mother pumps directly into the baby, eliminating the "middle man".

2. This means that the mother and baby should first get help with breastfeeding (improve the latch, use breast compression, switch sides), and when a baby truly needs supplementation, the supplement should be given at the breast with a lactation aid at the breast. Because:

- Breastfeeding is more than the milk and even if the mother is supplementing the baby with formula, supplementing the baby at the breast means the mother and baby are still breastfeeding. And if we may say it, breastfeeding *exclusively*, when we think of "breastfeeding" as a relationship. Do we say to couples unable to have children not to make love? Of course not! Because making love is about much more than making a baby.

- Babies learn to breastfeed *by breastfeeding.*

- Mothers learn to breastfeed *by breastfeeding.*

- The baby continues to get milk from the breast even as he is being supplemented.

- With supplementation *at the breast*, the milk supply increases.

- The baby is much less likely to reject the breast, refuse to latch on, in other words, than if he is supplemented by bottle. In fact, he will not reject the breast if the lactation aid is used properly with the baby having as good a latch as possible and the tube well placed. Other methods,

164

such supplementing with an open cup or finger feeding, though better than a bottle are still not methods of supplementation with the baby on the breast.

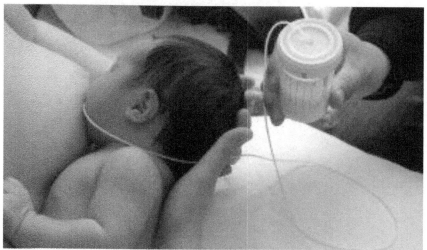

A baby being supplemented at the breast with a lactation aid. This method teaches a baby how to breastfeed, teaches the mother how to breastfeed, prevents breast rejection by the baby, allows the baby to continue getting milk from the breast even while being supplemented. This method also preserves breastfeeding which is much more than breastmilk.

The baby is not getting enough milk from the breast! What do we do now?

1.First of all, we help the mother and baby achieve the best latch possible. The better the latch, the more milk the baby will receive from the breast. Look at this baby at the breast (the photo below this paragraph). The latch is "asymmetric". Why is it better?

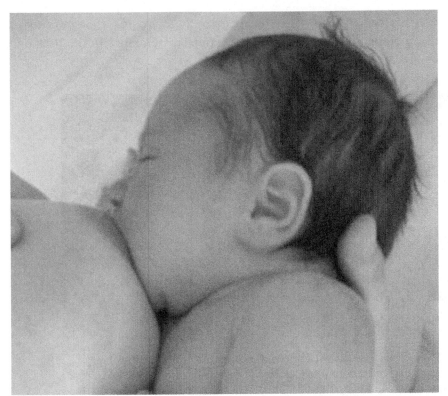

This baby has an asymmetric latch, – the chin is in breast, but the nose is not. He covers more of the areola with his lower lip than his upper lip and thus more of the breast is above/over the baby's lower jaw.

All of us who discuss breastfeeding, emphasize the importance of getting more of the breast into the baby's mouth. And an asymmetric latch gets more of the breast into the baby's mouth, at least more of the breast *where the baby's lower jaw is*. The baby is thus able to stimulate the release of milk from the breast better because of the sucking movements of the lower jaw. Compare with this baby's latch (photo under this paragraph):

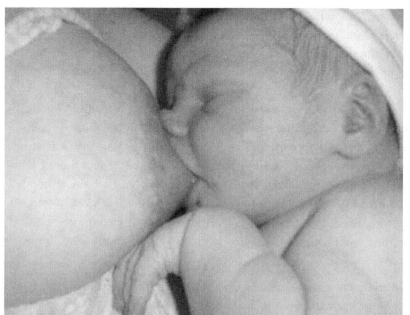

*This baby has a poor latch – the opposite of an asymmetric latch. The nose is in the breast, the chin is not. Compare his latch with the photo above this one. There is more breast under the baby's **upper lip and gums** than above the lower lip and gums and **tongue**. The maxilla (upper jaw) does not move and thus, does not stimulate the breast well enough to release milk from the breast.*

This baby's latch in the photo above is asymmetric alright, could be called a "reverse asymmetric latch". Compare the way this baby is latched on, to the way the other baby is latched on in the previous photo. In other words, the baby covers more of the areola with his upper lip than the lower lip. The part of the mouth that is supposed to stimulate the breast to release milk is a part of the mouth that *doesn't move,* so cannot truly stimulate the breast to release its milk as easily as it should. And where is the baby's tongue which also does a lot of the stimulation to release the milk? Right on the nipple, which can cause the mother nipple pain.

2. Once the mother has the baby latched on as well as possible, we show her how to know the baby is getting milk. How do we know the baby is getting milk? *Watch a video on www.ibconline.ca which shows a baby is drinking very*

167

well at the breast. The pause as he opens his mouth to the maximum is a sign that his mouth is filling with milk. The longer the pause, the more milk the baby received. As long as the baby is drinking like this, there is no need to use breast compression, *or take the baby off the breast or offer the other breast.*

It is for this reason "just feed the baby on one breast at each feeding" or "do block feeding" ("block feeding" involves feeding the baby on the same breast several feedings in a row before changing to the other breast and then feeding the baby on that breast several feedings in a row) so the baby gets more high fat milk is likely to cause late onset decreased milk supply. If a baby is not *drinking* at the breast, the baby is not getting high fat milk. He's getting no milk, low fat or high fat or intermediate fat. And persistent feeding on just one breast at a feeding will inevitably lead to a decrease in milk supply and milk flow to the baby.

3. Thus, when the baby is not drinking very much at the breast any longer, we recommend the mother start breast compressions.

Watch a video on www.ibconline.ca which shows how breast compressions help this 4 day old baby receive more milk. When a baby is sucking but not drinking much, the mother starts to compress her breast, with the result that the baby gets more milk. The mother compresses the breast and maintains the compression steady as long as the baby drinks. She then releases the compression. She waits to see if the baby starts to drink again, which occurs when the baby starts to taste milk again (babies respond to milk flow). If the baby sucks but does not drink, the mother repeats the compression, and so on until the baby hardly drinks.

4. When breast compressions no longer seem to get the baby more milk, the mother should offer the baby the other breast and repeat steps 1 to 3. If the baby is not getting as much milk has would have liked, he should be happy to take the second side. The problem is that many mothers will keep the baby on the one breast until the baby is fast asleep. If he is fast asleep, he may not wake up to take the second side even if he would take more milk. To illustrate: imagine a baby who has received 80% of the amount of milk he needs on the first breast. If he fast asleep on the first breast, he may not wake up right away

to take the other breast and the mother may feel he has finished. Consistently feeding on one breast only, following a "rule" may eventually lead to a decrease in milk supply.

The next two steps depend on the clinical situation. Neither may be necessary, and in fact for some babies, neither was necessary. Steps 1 to 4 were followed, and the baby started gaining weight without any galactagogues or supplementation used. He just got more and more milk as the mother's milk supply increased with a better latch and breast compressions.

Watch a video on www.ibconline.ca which shows a two week old baby with "borderline drinking". "Borderline" because there may not be enough drinking for the baby to gain weight well, but the baby is drinking enough so that the baby will not get ill or into trouble. In fact, the baby did very well without galactagogues (drugs/herbs that increase milk supply) or supplementation.

On the other hand, in some cases supplementation, discussed already, will still be necessary and if so, should be given on the second breast after the baby is no longer receiving much milk on that side, but again, before the baby is too sleepy. If the baby is very sleepy, inserting the lactation aid may result in the baby slipping down on the breast, possibly causing the mother pain, or slipping off the breast completely. It is better to insert the lactation aid too early than too late.

Watch a video on www.ibconline.ca which shows how to insert a lactation aid. But more importantly, it shows that babies respond to milk flow. When the flow slows, the baby tends to fall asleep at the breast. When flow is increased, in this case with a lactation aid at the breast, the baby wakes up and sucks vigorously.

Domperidone for the mother

5. In some cases, starting the mother on domperidone may be help, *along with steps 1 to 4,* to get the baby gaining weight well. We start with 30 mg (3 ten mg tablets) 3 times a day of domperidone and sometimes go up from there in two steps, first to 40 mg (4 tablets) 3 times a day and then 40 mg (4 tablets) 4 times

a day, or 6 tablets, 5 tablets, 5 tablets (total 16 tables) for convenience. Taking pills 3 times a day is easier than taking them 4 times a day. One 10 mg tablet 3 times a day as many physicians prescribe is actually rather useless for the majority of mothers. What's the point of prescribing a useless dose of a medication?

Domperidone is one of the safer medications around. The warning (in January 2015) by Health Canada is not based on good evidence and there is no good evidence there is a risk for any cardiac side effect with domperidone. (In fact, it is not a Health Canada warning, but rather an endorsed warning which originates from a company that makes domperidone). It is bizarre that the fax sent out by Health Canada in January 2015 does not mention any references though apparently this is not rare for Health Canada.

The warning is a word for word repetition of the statement by the European Medications Agency which gets many of its ideas from the drug manufacturers and formula companies. In spite of several deaths in Europe in mothers taking the birth control pill (and in Canada too – 23 deaths in 8 years in Canada as reported by Health Canada), everyone says that the birth control pill is worth the risk. Well, considering there are methods of contraception other than the birth control pill we would dispute that. But of course, the birth control pill is very much popular with physicians and other health professionals and pharmaceutical companies make a lot of money on the birth control pill, which is not the case with domperidone.

We checked with Health Canada in 2012 when all this hullabaloo started about domperidone in Canada. Health Canada had *never* received a report of a death in a breastfeeding woman that could be definitely attributed to her taking domperidone. We checked again after the January 2015 warning. No reports of any deaths that could definitely be attributed to domperidone in the age group of breastfeeding mothers. In fact, they have not had any reports of any significant side effects that can *definitely* be attributed to domperidone in patients of any age. Furthermore, we personally have treated tens of thousands of mothers with domperidone in much larger doses than Health Canada's recommended maximum dose and have recommended it for many more who then received a prescription from their own family doctor. Very few mothers had any side effects at all and those who did had very minor, transient ones that disappeared within days of starting the domperidone. In one study based on 1000 mother and baby pairs from our clinic (though we did not do the review), the Clinical Pharmacology Department of the Hospital for Sick Children found side effects in the mothers to be uncommon, mild and transient. The most common side effect was mild and transient headache lasting no more than a couple of days. There were not side effects noted in the baby. At the writing the study has been submitted for publication but not yet published.

How long do we recommend domperidone? We now encourage mothers to keep taking the domperidone until the baby is well established on food. That way, if the milk supply decreases when the mother decreases the dose of domperidone, which it does sometimes, the baby can make up the extra calories and nutrients he needs by eating more food until the mother can bump up the domperidone again. See also the website information sheets on domperidone including the one on stopping domperidone. See also the next chapter which is a more complete discussion on domperidone. We generally recommend dropping 1 pill per day a week, always on the same day of the week, so if the mother is taking 12 pills a day now, she will take 11 pills a day for a week, then one week later 10 pills a day for a week etc.

In some situations, it is not necessary to keep taking the domperidone. For example, we often use domperidone for a mother whose baby is not latching on. Even if the mother is expressing all the milk the baby needs, we believe that more milk means faster flow and faster flow means the baby is more likely to latch on. Once the baby is latched on, our experience shows that most mothers no longer need domperidone when the baby is latched on well. In this situation, the mother can wean off the domperidone more quickly and before the baby is taking solids.

What about the side effects we hear about when stopping domperidone?

Although very few of our own patients have ever complained of significant side effects when stopping domperidone slowly as we recommend, there are discussions on the internet about depression, sleeplessness and anxiety associated with stopping domperidone, almost always when it is stopped too quickly and when associated with stopping breastfeeding as well. So, stopping slowly, one pill a week (see above) is better than stopping quickly. Even if the mother is no longer breastfeeding, weaning from domperidone should be slow.

DOMPERIDONE

Domperidone can be very useful to increase the mother's milk supply and, more importantly, milk flow from the mother to the baby.

An important point: If all mothers had had the best start with **breastfeeding,** *from the very start,* **having as few interventions as is reasonable during** labour and birth **and the mothers and babies had received** good help from the beginning, **most mothers taking domperidone would not have needed it.**

In our clinic, we use domperidone for several reasons in addition to the situation when the baby is not getting enough milk from the breast and is already being supplemented with formula and with bottles.

For example, we sometimes use domperidone also when the baby is not latching on even if the mother is able to produce all the milk the baby needs, because increased milk production results, usually, in an increased milk flow and if there is increased milk flow the baby is more likely to latch on. A baby's beginning to latch on largely depends on milk flow from the breast.

We use it sometimes also when the mother has sore nipples because when the flow of milk is slow, a baby tends to slip down on to the nipple causing more pain and some babies will pull at the breast when the flow of milk is slow. As well, more milk means the baby will spend less time on the breast receiving more milk and will stay full longer with the result that the mother will get a longer break with the baby more satisfied.

We use it frequently when the mother has had late onset decreased milk supply. Incidentally, "decreased milk supply does not necessarily mean "not enough milk". Mothers who have had late onset decreased milk supply usually started out with an abundant milk supply, so "decreased" can still mean the baby is getting enough. However, the baby's behaviour shows that he is not happy with the flow of milk.

Late onset decreased milk supply is often, but by no means always, due to the **baby's having a tongue tie**. Releasing a tongue tie in the 3 or 4 month old baby, when the milk flow has decreased, sometimes results in the baby refusing the breast. Therefore, we prefer increasing the milk supply and flow *first* and then, a week or so later, releasing the tongue tie. There are other reasons for late onset decreased milk supply, such as **feeding one breast at a feeding** without offering the other, starting **hormonal birth control**, including intrauterine devices that release progestins, etc.

How does domperidone work?

Domperidone works by blocking dopamine at the periphery (*but not in the brain*) so that prolactin secretion by the pituitary gland is increased (dopamine inhibits the release of prolactin).

Many people seem to worry about blocking dopamine and what effect it may have on the functions of dopamine on mood; however, domperidone acts peripherally, *outside the brain*. According to Thomas Hale (author of *Medications and Mothers' Milk*) in a letter to the European Medications Agency, "Due to its unique structure, domperidone has very limited penetration of the blood-brain barrier. The central/peripheral ratio for domperidone is approximately 1:300, compared with 1:45 for metoclopramide, a similar drug. This, in practice, means a *very low incidence of CNS side effects in patients*." In other words, domperidone barely enters into the brain (does not pass the blood-brain barrier, the pituitary being "functionally" outside the blood brain-barrier).

By increasing the prolactin secretion from the pituitary, domperidone increases milk production and increases milk flow to the baby. And babies learn to breastfeed *by breastfeeding*. In other words, by getting milk from the breast (another reason to use the **lactation aid at the breast**, incidentally).

But domperidone must not be used in isolation. It is also important to **improve the baby's latch** and also use **breast compression** to increase the flow of milk to the baby. And to make sure the baby is **fed on both breasts** at each feeding.

And if supplementation is required, using a lactation aid at the breast works better than any type of supplementation away from the breast (bottle, cup, finger feeding, nipple shield). Domperidone is important, while at the same time not the only approach for the baby not getting enough milk from the breast.

Does domperidone work for everyone?

No drug works for everyone in every situation or in the same way for different people, whether it be a drug for high blood pressure, an antibiotic to treat pneumonia, or any drug for any problem. In this, domperidone is not different from other drugs.

But there are ways to improve the likelihood that domperidone will work. A major problem interfering with domperidone's action is the use of bottles to supplement the baby. Bottles interfere with how a baby latches on and thus decrease the effect of domperidone. Improving the latch and using breast compression are helpful to get the better results from domperidone. Using a lactation aid at the breast to supplement instead of a bottle also increases the likelihood that domperidone will work better. In other words, domperidone is not a magic bullet and is only part of the approach to increasing milk intake by the baby.

Is domperidone safe?

In fact, domperidone is one of the safer medications around. True, there is no such thing as a drug that has no side effects, including serious ones, and domperidone has some as well. As Hale has written in the same document as above: "At a minimum, more than a billion doses have been used in Europe alone and many more world-wide, in perhaps millions of patients".

"...Domperidone has an excellent safety profile and is generally very well tolerated."

A recent study in our clinic patients, done on the records of 1000 mothers and their babies by the department of clinical pharmacology of the Hospital for Sick

Children, showed very few side effects. The most common (in 10% of mothers) was *mild* and *transient* headache. Also reported, but not seen in this study, is weight gain in about 10% of mothers. Incidentally, this study suggested that the use of domperidone increased the mother's production of milk by 28%. Other studies have shown an increase in milk production by the mother of up to 96%.

The warnings (in 2012 and 2015) by Health Canada are not based on good evidence and there is no good evidence at all that there is a risk from any cardiac side effect with domperidone. (In fact, it is not a Health Canada warning at all, but rather an endorsed warning which originates from a company that makes domperidone, attempting to covering their liability). It is bizarre that the fax sent out by Health Canada in January 2015 does not mention any references though apparently this is not rare for Health Canada. Even someone who has a prolonged QT interval, well, in theory there is a risk, but in practical terms there is probably not.

Health Canada's warning is a word for word repetition of the statement by the European Medications Agency which gets many of its ideas from the drug manufacturers and formula companies. In spite of several deaths in Europe in mothers taking the birth control pill (and in Canada too: 23 deaths in 8 years in Canada as reported by **Health Canada in 2013**), everyone seems to agree that the birth control pill is worth the risk. Well, considering there are methods of contraception other than the birth control pill, including the **lactation amenorrhea method (LAM)** in breastfeeding mothers, we would dispute that. But of course, the birth control pill is very popular with physicians and other health professionals and the pharmaceutical companies make a lot of money on the birth control pill, which is not the case with domperidone. We checked with Health Canada in 2012 when all this started about domperidone in Canada. Health Canada has never had a report of an unexpected death in a breastfeeding woman taking domperidone. We checked again after the January 2015 warning. No reports of any deaths in the age group of mothers breastfeeding. In fact, they have not had any reports of any significant side effects that can *definitely* be attributed to domperidone *in patients of any age.*

However, almost all drugs have caused death, one way or another. The birth control pill has already been mentioned. Used even more frequently, antibiotics, amongst the most commonly used drugs, have caused death in several ways, occasionally causing a very serious skin disease called Stevens-Johnson syndrome (or toxic epidermal necrolysis) which has a high death rate. Antibiotics may also cause an infection of the gut with a bacterium called *C. difficile*. This infection is not uncommon at all and severe illness and even death from this infection are reported several times every year.

I have personally treated many thousands of mothers with domperidone in much larger doses than Health Canada's recommended maximum dose and have recommended it for many more who then received a prescription from their own family doctor. Very few mothers had any side effects at all and those who did had very minor ones that disappeared within days.

This is not to say that we should use medication lightly without consideration of the possible side effects. Still, if breastfeeding is important, as we believe it is, use of domperidone can be very helpful.

Here is an **editorial in the British Medical Journal** about an increased risk of venous thromboembolism (potentially fatal) with the newer versions of the birth control pill.

This is the difference between domperidone and the birth control pill: When a study finds that birth control pills cause a much higher rate of venous thromboembolism (as discussed in this editorial), one only needs to scroll down on the commentary to read the following:

"These results ... provide important guidance for the safe prescribing of oral contraceptives."

What does this mean? We can use birth control pills cautiously but without worry because the benefit outweighs the risk. On the other hand, we can't use domperidone because improving breastfeeding success is not important.

There are so many much more dangerous drugs out there than domperidone. The same worries about a prolonged QT interval could be voiced about many drugs that are used daily, including some antibiotics, but the current discussion seems to single out domperidone only. Why would that be? Again, because improving breastfeeding is of no real importance, since we have such **wonderful breastmilk substitutes; NOT**.

Indeed, metoclopramide which is commonly used in the US instead of domperidone to increase milk supply has been associated with permanent neurological dysfunction and has been getting none of the negative publicity in spite of a **black box warning on metoclopramide** by the US Federal Drug Administration.

And what about acetaminophen? Yes, that stuff that parents give to their children every time they have a fever or an ache or a pain? Read the **article on the Huffington Post** and this, in the article: "Acetaminophen overdose sends as many as 78,000 Americans to the emergency room annually and results in 33,000 hospitalizations a year, federal data shows. Acetaminophen is also the nation's leading cause of acute liver failure, according to data from an ongoing study funded by the National Institutes for Health."

So, what is all this fuss about domperidone?

Exactly, what is all the fuss about?

I receive emails from mothers who say that, according to their doctor, they cannot take domperidone because they had a murmur when they were children or because their grandfather had a heart attack or because they had an operation for a hole in the heart when they were babies or because they occasionally have palpitations and other completely irrelevant issues. The *only* reason for concern is if the mother has a prolonged QT interval on electrocardiogram and this problem is very uncommon if not rare in a population of women of reproductive age. This one uncommon indication has been widened to include every possible heart problem that one can imagine.

In a recently published protocol on galactogogues, the Academy of Breastfeeding Medicine, bizarrely, added "a high BMI" (a sign of overweight) to the contraindications for the use of domperidone.

The situation is bizarre. A mother going to the pharmacy with a prescription for domperidone may be asked for what reason she will be taking domperidone. If she answers, "for increasing my milk supply", she will be told in many pharmacies that her prescription for domperidone cannot be filled. If she answers, "for gastric problems", she will be told, "Oh, your prescription will be ready in 15 to 20 minutes. We will call you on this beeper when it's ready."

That's it! According to the strange thinking of the European Medications Agency and the copycat thinking of Health Canada, domperidone is dangerous only if you are taking it to improve breastfeeding, but not to deal with gastric problems.

But, here is a secret. The European Medications Agency's own studies showed no effect on QT interval in healthy volunteers.

After all is said and done, if you have unexplained palpitations or a significant family history of unexpected cardiac arrest, have an electrocardiogram, with special attention to a prolonged QT interval, before starting the domperidone.

What is the dose of domperidone?

We start with a dose of 30 mg (3 tablets, as the only available size of a tablet is 10 mg) of domperidone 3 times a day. We then *might* increase the dose in two steps, if the response to the lower dose is not as good as it could be, first to 40 (4 tablets) 3 times a day and then 16 tablets a day, divided into three doses (6 tablets, 5 tablets, 5 tablets, for a total of 16).

The reason for going up in 2 steps is basically to find the lowest dose that actually works, taking into consideration that the higher the dose of *any* drug, the more likely there will be side effects.

179

On the recommendation of Health Canada, mothers are often treated with only 10 mg (1 tablet) 3 times a day. A small number of mothers do seem to get an effect from this tiny dose, but we believe that helping the mother improve the breastfeeding with **a better latch** and using **breast compression** would have prevented the "need" for domperidone in mothers who respond to 10 mg three times a day. Furthermore, it is strange to worry about the side effects of a drug but then prescribe an inadequate, usually useless, dose.

How long should the mother take the domperidone?

We now encourage mothers to keep taking the domperidone until the baby is well established on **food**). That way, if the milk supply decreases when the mother decreases the dose of domperidone, the baby can make up the extra calories and nutrients he needs by **eating more food** until the dose of domperidone can be bumped up again.

But this is not always necessary by any means. If the domperidone is used to increase the flow so that the baby who is not latching on is encouraged to latch on, then once the baby is latched on and drinking well, the mother can wean off the domperidone (more quickly than as described below), as a baby well latched on can get more milk from the breast than a pump.

How to wean off the domperidone

We generally recommend dropping 1 pill per day a week, always on the same day of the week, so if the mother is taking 12 pills a day now, next week, she will take 11 pills a day for a week, then one week later 10 pills a day etc. In other words, it will take 12 weeks to wean off the domperidone completely.

The reason for slowly weaning off the domperidone is that there are reports that rapid weaning off the domperidone after the mother has been taking it for several months may lead to symptoms of anxiety, sleeplessness and depression in the mother. This does not seem to have been a common problem amongst our patients, as they tend to follow our approach of slow weaning off the domperidone.

Is this syndrome of anxiety due somehow to domperidone? Probably it is due to rapid decrease in the prolactin levels, which are also seen in mothers who stop breastfeeding "cold turkey" and also women who are treated with drugs such as cabergoline which decrease prolactin levels.

What people often ask about is the effect on the baby

As with almost all medications, the amount of domperidone that enters the milk is minuscule and very unlikely to cause any problems for the baby. If the mother is taking 80 mg of domperidone a day, the amount the baby would get in the milk is 0.007 micrograms (nothing to do with James Bond), an insignificant, minuscule dose. Furthermore, domperidone actually is not well absorbed from the stomach and intestinal tract, and only about 15% of the ingested dose is actually absorbed. So, side effects or harm to the baby is vanishingly small, in fact zero.

Anything else?

It has been suggested that domperidone only releases stored prolactin from the pituitary gland and once the prolactin has been released, the effect of domperidone wears off. We do see that some of our patients get an initial good response to domperidone, but it does not last and declines after 3 or 4 days to a week. But the explanation of depletion of prolactin from the pituitary just does not make sense.

First of all, because it certainly does seem to occur, but only in a very small minority of mothers.

Secondly, because when this does occur, increasing the dose of domperidone will overcome this decline in the effect of the domperidone. Thus, some prolactin is left in the pituitary? What's the explanation? We don't know.

MATERNAL MEDICATIONS AND BREASTFEEDING

Here is one of the most common breastfeeding questions we receive: "I have been put on such and such drug and have been told I cannot breastfeed. Is that true?"

The short answer is: **Almost no medication taken by the mother requires her to stop or interrupt breastfeeding.** The real question, though, is "Which is safer for the baby? Breastfeeding with *minuscule* amounts of drug in the milk, (and the amounts in the milk are almost always minuscule), or artificial feeding?" The answer is, *with very few exceptions*, "keep breastfeeding, it's better for your baby and also for you, the mother".

This is true, in spite of doctors telling mothers they cannot breastfeed because there are no studies that have been done on most drugs and breastfeeding. This response is a complete cop-out. Telling the mother that there are no studies on a particular drug and breastfeeding usually is not true. Often there *are* studies, but usually only *on small numbers of mothers and babies*. The doctor giving this answer is a handy, plausible way for the physician or pharmacist to tell the mother that she cannot breastfeed. There are ways, however, of deciding if a drug taken by the mother is compatible with continued breastfeeding. Good studies, on more than a handful of breastfeeding mothers and babies, are nice to have, but not always necessary.

In fact, there is good, scientific information, very useful information, with regard to the majority of drugs. And the information available makes it possible, in the vast majority of cases, to be able to say to a mother: "Yes, keep breastfeeding, it is best for the baby and for you". A good text is Medications and Mother's Milk, by Thomas Hale. You can find out by sending me your question. As mentioned above, however, the real question is: which is safer for the baby: breastfeeding with minuscule amounts of drug in the milk or artificial feeding? After all is said and done, breastfeeding is almost always safer, not only for the baby, but also for the mother.

Why is continuing breastfeeding almost always safer for the baby?

The reason is that big little word "minuscule". With the vast majority of drugs, so little of the medication enters the mother's milk, that when one compares the risks of not breastfeeding to the risk, almost non-existent, of that tiny amount of drug in the milk, it is clear that continuing breastfeeding is safer for the baby and for the mother.

Whereas minuscule amounts of drug getting into the milk only rarely have any risks for the baby, the risks of *not* breastfeeding are well documented, not only for the baby, but also for the mother, so the risks for the mother also need also to be taken into account. Which risks? Of course, there is the risk of painful engorgement and mastitis despite pumping. But we are talking long term: a mother who breastfeeds has a lower risk of **breast cancer, ovarian cancer** and likely uterine cancer. As well, she has a lower risk of **high blood pressure, high cholesterol, and insulin resistance**. *And the longer the mother breastfeeds, the lower her risks.*

When it is a **toddler at the breast**, another issue arises. Many toddlers are very attached to breastfeeding, and whether one agrees with toddlers breastfeeding or not (actually, what is wrong with it?), forcing the toddler from the breast can result in serious and **prolonged emotional distress.** Any mother who has been faced with a "need" to stop breastfeeding an 18 month old, and trying to do so, knows that this is true.

Why are the amounts of most drugs in the milk so low?

The amount of any drug that gets into the milk depends first and foremost on *the drug being in the blood.* If the drug is not in the blood, it cannot get into the milk.

This is important when mothers are told that they cannot breastfeed if they are using eye drops, for example. How much drug could get into the blood since the cornea of the eye has no blood supply? The minimal amount in contact with the conjunctiva or that goes down the tear ducts into the mother's mouth?

That is ridiculous. It is the same for tooth whitener as the enamel of the teeth has no blood supply. We receive a surprising number of emails asking about tooth whiteners.

A drug that is not absorbed into the mother's blood from her intestines or elsewhere also cannot get into the milk. A few examples of drugs not getting into the blood from "elsewhere".

1. Botox is a perfect example and one of the common questions we get. Botox stays where it is injected, otherwise it would be of no use and would be dangerous to the mother. It doesn't get into the blood, so cannot get into the milk.

2. Drugs that are used to treat varicose veins are another group of drugs we hear about all the time. Typically, mothers are told they must not breastfeed after these highly irritating chemicals are injected into the veins. However, for these medications to be effective, they are intended to stay at the injection site. If they got into the general circulation, the problem would be for the mother because of how irritating these chemicals are. But they don't get into the general circulation, so they cannot get into the milk.

So what information is available to help decide if a drug gets into the milk?

1. In some cases, a drug does not get into the milk at all, the amounts are zero. Here are some examples:

• Monoclonal antibodies such as etanercept (Enbrel) and infliximab (Remicade) and many newer ones, are now commonly used to treat inflammatory and other diseases such as multiple sclerosis, psoriasis, rheumatoid arthritis, Crohn's disease, asthma, and many others thought to be due to an abnormal immune response. These monoclonal antibodies, also called "biologicals", are, essentially, antibodies and as such are very large molecules with a molecular weight of approximately 150,000 Daltons. Any drug having a molecular weight of 600 to 800 or more Daltons is *too large to get into the milk*.

• Heparin is a drug used to prevent clotting of the blood, an anticoagulant. It is too large to get into the milk. Even "low molecular weight" heparin with a molecular weight of 4500, is only "low molecular weight" compared to regular heparin with a molecular weight of 15,000.

• Interferons, used for many illnesses, including multiple sclerosis, have a molecular weight of between 20,000 and 30,000. **Too large to get into the milk**. Another drug commonly used for **multiple sclerosis** is glatiramer (Copaxone), which also does not get into the milk because the molecule weight is too big. In addition, glatiramer is not absorbed from the intestinal tract, so even if, by some unusual circumstance, it did get into the milk, it would end up in the baby's diaper.

• Luteinizing hormone and follicle stimulating hormone frequently used to induce ovulation, have molecular weights in the thousands, too large to get into the milk.

2. An important factor determining how much of a drug gets into the milk is how much of the drug is bound to protein. Only drug that is *not* attached to protein can get into the milk; only the "free" drug can get into the milk. Below is a random list of commonly used drugs that are very highly protein bound:

• Ketorolac (Toradol): 99% of the drug in the mother's blood is bound to protein, so only 1% of the already tiny amount of drug in the mother's blood can actually get into the milk. Ibuprofen (Advil) is more than 99% bound to protein. Meloxicam (Mobic) is >99% protein bound. Diclofenac (Voltaren) is 99.7% protein bound. In fact, as with the above examples, most of the nonsteroidal anti-inflammatory drugs (NSAIDs), have similar protein binding.

• Others: warfarin (Coumadin), an anticoagulant (99% protein bound), diazepam, an anti-anxiety medication (99% protein bound), propranolol a beta-blocker used to treat high blood pressure, migraines, the symptoms of overactive thyroid amongst other problems (90% protein bound).

Warfarin has been used for decades to prevent blood clotting and if the patient's prothrombin time (a measure of how easily the patient bleeds) is

185

followed and kept within a certain range, it is safe for the patient. And safe for the baby.

But here is a perfect example of how doctors do not consider breastfeeding important or consider it at all when they prescribe for breastfeeding mothers. There are several new medications to prevent clotting. And doctors love new medications. They too often believe the "hype" from the drug company representatives and advertisements and then a few years later it is sometimes found not to be as safe for the adult as the doctors were told. But instead of prescribing warfarin for the mother and following the prothrombin time, they prescribe the new medication and tell the mother she has to stop breastfeeding because "there are no studies" available. Maybe the mother would prefer to have her prothrombin levels followed, even if that required having blood taken at regular intervals, if that allowed her to continue breastfeeding.

3. Many drugs given to mothers may get into their milk, but the baby will not absorb the drug and thus such a drug should be safe during breastfeeding.

• A special situation is that of the *proton pump inhibitors*, used by millions of people to treat gastro-esophageal reflux disease (GERD); for example, pantoprazole (Tecta) and lansoprazole (Prevacid). This family of drugs are immediately destroyed by stomach acid, but, because they have a protective covering, they are protected from destruction in the mother's stomach and are well absorbed by the mother. However, whatever drug gets into the milk (and that is a minuscule amount, as is typical), no longer has the protective covering and is destroyed in the baby's stomach. If you are taking such a drug, check the label on the container. It will usually say something like "Do not break, chew, or crush". Why? If the protective covering of the drug is disrupted, the drug will be destroyed in the *mother's* stomach.

• Several antibiotics may get into the milk but are not absorbed by the baby. Gentamicin and tobramycin are in the family of antibiotics called aminoglycosides. Vancomycin is another drug that may get into the milk in tiny amounts but is not absorbed from the baby's intestinal tract. The absorption of these drugs from the gut is essentially zero. Thus, whatever tiny amount of the drug gets into the milk will end up in the baby's diaper.

186

Some will argue that the antibiotic may cause a change in the baby's microbiome (intestinal flora), but then if the mother is told she cannot breastfeed and gives the baby formula, then the baby's microbiome will change as well because the baby is fed formula. Is it better to change the microbiome with formula? No! Because at the same time we are interrupting breastfeeding and a week or 10 days without breastfeeding is almost surely going to be the end of breastfeeding.

Mothers have also been told that the baby may become allergic to the antibiotic. That is highly unlikely. Besides, doctors are rarely held back from prescribing antibiotics for babies, far too often for illnesses that don't require antibiotics. And if the baby goes on formula, the baby may become allergic to components of the formula.

• Another interesting example is tetracycline, a broad-spectrum antibiotic taken these days mostly for the treatment of acne. Everyone seems to believe that tetracycline is contraindicated during breastfeeding because it is contraindicated during pregnancy *and* in children under the age of 8 years (some say 12 years) due to discolouration and weakness it can cause in developing teeth and bones. But the pharmacist will tell you *not* to take tetracycline with milk. Why? Because tetracycline combines with calcium in the milk and is not absorbed. If the breastfeeding mother is taking tetracycline, how will the baby get the tetracycline? With milk! And so the tetracycline ends up in the baby's diaper not in his bones and teeth.

What about doxycycline, related to tetracycline, used not infrequently these days for Lyme disease, malaria prophylaxis, treatment of acne and rosacea and several other reasons. Is it contraindicated during breastfeeding? **It is not contraindicated during breastfeeding**, though some experts recommend limiting treatment to 3 to 6 weeks which may be a problem for mothers taking it for acne or rosacea, since that requires long term treatment. The concern is doxycycline decreasing the calcium intake of the baby and resulting calcium deficiency. Though this seems unlikely with the minuscule amount of doxycycline that gets into the milk, if it is necessary to treat longer term, the baby can be given extra calcium.

4. Many drugs result in very low blood levels in the mother's blood because the majority of the drug is elsewhere in her body than in her blood. This is indicated by the measurement called "volume of distribution" of the drug. The larger the volume of distribution of a drug, the less likely the drug is to be in the mother's blood, or, said in another way, the lower the concentration in the blood. For example, most of the antidepressants like sertraline (Zoloft), citalopram (Celexa), and most others in the same family of drugs, naturally reside in the brain where they affect the mother's mood and are not in the blood except in minuscule amounts.

5. Many drugs have poor absorption from the baby's intestinal tract, so that even if some drug gets into the milk, very little will be absorbed into the baby's blood.

Propranolol, mentioned above as having 90% protein binding, is an example of how we can put two or more pieces of information together, even if "not enough studies have been done". In addition to the high protein binding of propranolol, we also know that only about 30% of the propranolol in the intestines is actually absorbed into the body, not only for the mother but also for the baby. Furthermore, we know that there is very little propranolol circulating in the mother's blood. So, is propranolol safe to take during breastfeeding? Yes!

Nitrendipine (Baypress), a drug used for hypertension? 98% protein bound, and oral absorption of less than 20%. Nifedipine, in the same family of drugs as Nitrendipine, is 92 to 98% protein bound, and oral absorption from the intestinal tract is 50%. Both safe.

Other drugs? The monoclonal antibodies (mentioned in point 1.) also do not get absorbed from the intestinal tract at all as they are almost surely completely destroyed in the baby's stomach. Furthermore, even if, by some fluke, they got pas the stomach, they would not be absorbed by the baby and end up in the diaper. But monoclonal antibodies don't get into the milk in the first place.

Corticosteroids

Mothers are not infrequently treated with corticosteroids (prednisone, prednisolone and other forms intravenously) for autoimmune diseases, for asthma, poison ivy and many other reasons. Corticosteroids can be given orally, intravenously for illnesses such as multiple sclerosis, ulcerative colitis, into the joints for inflammatory illnesses of the joints, and for many other reasons, including during pregnancy to prevent the baby from having breathing difficulties after birth when the baby risks being born prematurely.

As with other medications mentioned here, the blood levels are very low and the milk levels consequently very low. When injected into a joint, the corticosteroids stay in the joint, they stay put and don't get into the mother's blood; therefore, they cannot get into the milk. Moreover, when pregnant women are given corticosteroids if premature birth is threatened, they are not made to worry about it in the same way breastfeeding mothers are.

Breastfeeding after general anesthetic

Mothers are usually told that they will have to interrupt breastfeeding for 24 to 48 hours after surgery under general anesthetic. Recently one mother who contacted me was told she would have to interrupt breastfeeding for 8 days after the surgery. This is completely unnecessary and extremely harmful to the mother (engorgement despite expression, decreased milk supply despite expression, baby refusing the breast; and having to deal with a crying, desperate baby who needs to breastfeed) and harmful to the baby as well (emotionally because of being denied the comfort and security of the breast, the possibility that the baby will refuse other forms of fluid and nutrition, ending up in hospital for rehydration). It is worth remembering that we frequently give babies having surgery the very same medication.

Two types of drugs are usually given during general anesthesia, some given by intravenous injection, usually to relax the patient, and/or to decrease lung secretions and, others to put the patient to sleep, as a gas given by mask or through a tube in the trachea. With regard to the drugs given by intravenous injection the issue is no different than any other drugs given by mouth or by injection. The concentration of the drugs in the mother's blood given by injection, especially intravenous injection, will rise quickly and then start to decrease very soon after the injection. With regard to breastfeeding, the concentration in the milk will remain low and will be very low or even absent by the time the mother wakes up.

As for the gas the mother inhales, well, the effects of the gas occur *by inhaling* it. Even if some entered the milk, the gas has no effect in the baby's stomach. It must be inhaled.

The bottom line? The mother can and should breastfeed as soon as she is awake and alert enough not to be afraid to drop the baby. If the mother is alert, the drugs have essentially left her body and no longer get into the milk, if they ever did get into the milk.

Some other drugs

1. Alcohol. Alcohol is *not* different from most other drugs in that very little gets into the milk. It is very different in that there is a level of paranoia amongst certain persons who state that even 1 drop of alcohol ingested by the baby is poison and dangerous. This is absurd.

The reasons for which people drink alcohol are complex, but in general, people, including breastfeeding mothers, drink alcoholic beverages for the effect the alcohol has on their mood. People, including breastfeeding mothers, enjoy the relaxation effect that small, reasonable amounts of alcohol have, and the "social lubricant" that alcohol causes in a gathering of people.

Alcohol is also special from the point of view of breastfeeding in that it moves back and forth between blood and milk and then back again from the milk to the blood as if it were water, which means that as the alcohol blood level decreases (as it does if the mother does not drink more), the alcohol in the milk will move back into the blood to "even out" the levels. This means that the mother should not pump her milk "to get rid of the alcohol" because it does not make a difference. The levels of alcohol in the milk are so low that it is not helpful to pump out the milk. Why is it not helpful?

In most jurisdictions in North America, Australia and Europe, the amount of alcohol in the blood for a person to be considered too impaired to drive is 0.05% or, in some, 0.08%. Now, if the mother's blood contains 0.08% alcohol, so will her milk contain 0.08% alcohol. If one considers that de-alcoholised beer actually contains around 0.6% alcohol, almost 8 times more than 0.08% and more than 10 more than 0.05%, it is obvious that the concentration of alcohol in the mother's milk is negligible. And not going to harm the baby.

The problem is that in most families, it is true that it is the mother who cares for the baby most of the time, and in breastfeeding families this likely to be even more the case. A mother has to be able to take care of her baby without her judgment regarding the baby's needs being impaired. That's all. So, mothers should not drink so much that their judgement is impaired.

See this article: *Basic Clinical Pharmacology and Toxicology* **2014;114:168-173.** One conclusion: *"It appears biologically implausible that occasional exposure to such amounts should be related to clinically meaningful effects to the nursing children. The effect of occasional alcohol consumption on milk production is small, temporary and unlikely to be of clinical relevance. Generally, there is little clinical evidence to suggest that breastfed children are adversely affected in spite of the fact that almost half of all lactating women in Western countries ingest alcohol occasionally."*

Finally, there is no evidence that the baby getting insignificant amounts of alcohol in the milk will predispose the baby to abusing alcohol in later life.

2. What has been said about most drugs is also true about nicotine and caffeine. Very little gets into the milk. A study several years ago showed that a baby whose mother smokes, but also breastfeeds, is healthier than if the mother smokes and does not breastfeed. Of course, it would be best if the mother did not smoke at all, for her own health. As for caffeine, it is worth noting that we give caffeine, in much larger doses than would get into the milk, to premature babies to prevent apnea (stopping breathing).

3. Other recreational drugs. These drugs, for example, marijuana and cocaine, have the same negative associations as does alcohol and on top of that in most jurisdictions are illegal to possess. We are not recommending that anyone break the law. But what we have said about alcohol is true of these drugs as well. That is, if the mother is so impaired that she cannot make a good judgment about her baby's needs, that is potentially dangerous for the baby. For example, if the mother is high on marijuana and the baby becomes sick and is not improving, would the mother notice that the baby is sick? Would she get into her car and drive the baby to the doctor or the hospital while her judgment is impaired?

The tetrahydrocannabinol (THC), the compound in marijuana is very highly protein bound, 99.9% protein bound. Furthermore, if taken by mouth (as might the baby) it is very poorly absorbed from the intestinal tract with only 6 to 20% of it absorbed. With such high protein binding, it is unlikely that significant amounts will get into the milk. But note again, that the "high" the mother experiences could last for a few hours, and so her judgement will also be impaired.

Cannabidiol (CBD), is now used widely as treatment for various medical disorders (medical marijuana) and thus not really a drug of recreation. It has low oral absorption, less than 20% of the orally taken dose, is absorbed.

What if my doctor or pharmacist says I need to stop breastfeeding with a particular medication?

1. Unfortunately, most doctors, including pediatricians and obstetricians, and even pharmacists (yes, even pharmacists), if they even bothered checking what the manufacturer of the drug says in its prescribing information, would not get good information. Basically, all drug companies say that breastfeeding should not continue while taking the drug. Or, at best, the information that comes with the drug will say that the breastfeeding mother should check with her doctor. But the companies write this to cover their medical- legal liability. They don't give a damn about the mother and the baby. And what's the point of asking the doctor, since many doctors don't know the first thing about

maternal medications and breastfeeding and will agree with whatever the pharmaceutical company says? Which is, "check with your doctor"!?

2. But the truth is that many doctors don't bother to check even the poor information about the drug from the manufacturers and merely assume that any drug is contraindicated during breastfeeding. They may not think "Oh, I prescribed this same drug for the baby 2 weeks ago and I wasn't particularly worried about it."

3. In the rare case where a drug is truly of concern, usually there are alternatives that could be used instead. For example, a mother taking heparin during the pregnancy might opt to continue heparin after the baby is born in order to avoid a brand new oral anticoagulant about which little is know regarding its safety for the baby during breastfeeding. She might do this, so she can breastfeed her baby, in spite of the pain of injecting heparin.

Unfortunately, too many doctors base their decisions on which drugs to use on pharmaceutical company marketing (conferences where paid representatives of the companies tell them how wonderful such and such a drug is) and the pharmaceutical company representative that drops by the doctor's office for 30 minutes every few months to keep him up to date. Incidentally, warfarin, an oral anticoagulant which is still the most commonly used oral coagulant, is still okay to take while breastfeeding.

4. And why do so many physicians assume that any and every drug is contraindicated during breastfeeding? Basically, because they don't believe that it matters if the mother breastfeeds or not. **Formula=breastmilk, bottle feeding=breastfeeding**, it's all the same. But it's *not* all the same.

5. So, although there are definitely exceptions, most doctors are not to be believed about information they give about drugs and breastfeeding. A mother should take "You must take *this* drug and you cannot breastfeed while taking it" with a grain of salt and seek a reliable source for information. There is good information out there, but a mother needs to know how to find it.

Some medications can reduce the milk supply

Some medications can decrease the milk production. Some can increase the milk production, **domperidone** for example, so maybe it is not surprising that some may reduce the milk production.

What causes the milk supply to increase in the first few days after birth? It is the *rapid drop* in progesterone and estrogen from the high levels that are normal during pregnancy, after the baby and placenta are born. In some hospitals, particularly in the US, mothers have been routinely given an injection of a progesterone type hormone (Depo-Provera) often without the mothers being given the information that the injection might decrease the milk supply. And not unusually, at least in the past, without being told the injection is birth control. One hopes that the notion of "informed consent" has filtered down even to these institutions.

Any treatment of the breastfeeding mother with female hormones may decrease milk production. The most common situations include the mother being prescribed the birth control pill, either a combination of estrogen and progesterone or progesterone alone ("minipill").

Mothers are frequently told by obstetricians that these hormonal methods do not decrease milk production, but how would an obstetrician really know? In North America, the obstetrician will typically see the mother at the routine 6 week checkup after the birth and at that time will recommend either a birth control pill or an intrauterine device which releases progesterone. The mother will be told these methods are necessary because "they cannot count on breastfeeding to prevent pregnancy". So, the mother takes these medications and within a week or 10 days after starting the hormones, she finds that the baby is pulling at the breast, crying at the breast and obviously is not getting enough at the breast.

So how would the obstetrician know that hormones do not interfere with milk supply? It is unlikely the obstetrician will see the mother again, until the next pregnancy, if there is one, unless the mother is having some sort of problem related to the birth or some sort of gynecological problem. And will the

194

obstetrician ask how the breastfeeding went? Very unlikely, as most obstetricians are not interested in how the breastfeeding went.

There are methods of birth control that do not involve using hormones.

Lactation Amenorrhea Method

Yes, breastfeeding can prevent pregnancy. Breastfeeding prevents ovulation and thus pregnancy if the following conditions are met:

1. The baby is less than 6 months old and is breastfed exclusively.

2. Breastfeeding according to the baby's cues and without use of artificial nipples, including pacifiers.

3. The mother and baby spend their days and nights together and **the baby sleeps with the mother** and breastfeeds as he wishes.

4. The mother has not had a return of her menstrual cycle and has not observed signs of her fertility returning and she has been taught how to watch for these signs.

Once the baby has started eating food at around 6 months, the likelihood of the return of fertility is increased. At this time the mother should observe signs of her fertility returning, because it is conceivable (sorry!) that the mother might become pregnant during her first postpartum ovulation and thus before having a menstrual period.

The reliable sign fertility is presence of fertile cervical mucus that occurs around the time of ovulation.

Artificial methods of contraception

If the couple want to use some contraceptive method that does not interfere with milk production, then barrier methods (condoms) or an intrauterine device that does not release hormones can be used.

Other medications that can reduce the milk supply

Cabergoline (Dostinex) and bromocriptine (Parlodel) are two drugs that inhibit the secretion of prolactin and thus will diminish the production of milk. As far as we are concerned, these medications should be absolutely avoided in breastfeeding mothers.

In some countries in Europe these drugs are used to treat postpartum engorgement and mastitis. Neither of these reasons is an indication for the use of cabergoline or bromocriptine nor does this constitute good treatment of engorgement or mastitis. The treatment for **postpartum engorgement** is *prevention* and if it does occur, helping the baby latch on better and breastfeed better for the breasts to be better emptied, and also to relieve engorgement. The treatment for **mastitis** is the same: *prevention* and ensuring the best latch possible and if mastitis does occur, helping the baby breastfeed better and sometimes antibiotics.

Antihistamines, particularly the older ones such as diphenhydramine (Benadryl) do seem to decrease milk production, at least based on the experiences of our patients.

Antihistamines are present in oral "cold medications" and also in "allergy medications" and these should therefore be avoided as should drugs such as pseudoephedrine. What can be done for cold symptoms and allergic symptoms? Frequently, no medications are necessary to treat the symptoms of cold. If the mother does feel she needs to take something, we wonder why people need to drug their entire body when treating symptoms locally is not only safer but also more effective and less likely to decrease the milk supply.

1. Eye symptoms can be treated with antihistamine drops or vasoconstrictive drops or both. Cromolyn eye drops are also available though hardly ever prescribed these days. Generally, it is better to avoid corticosteroid eye drops as they can cause serious damage to the eye if used when a person has herpes simplex of the cornea. However, they do not pose a problem for the breastfed

baby. If corticosteroid eye drops are prescribed by an ophthalmologist, the mother can and should continue breastfeeding.

2. Rhinitis (runny nose, blocked nose) can be treated with vasoconstrictive drops, antihistamine drops, or steroid sprays or all three. Also, these drugs are not a problem for the breastfed baby.

3. Breathing difficulties can be treated with salbutamol spray or steroid inhalers or oral corticosteroids (prednisone, for example) if severe. And these drugs are also not a problem for the baby.

4. Skin problems (urticaria or hives) can also be treated with local antihistamine creams/ointments or a short course of oral corticosteroids rather than oral antihistamines. This is also true for problems such as poison ivy.

GASTROENTERITIS IN THE BREASTFED BABY

This article specifically discusses infection of the gastrointestinal tract because it is the most common acute infant illness that too many physicians and other health professionals insist requires the mothers to interrupt breastfeeding. Unfortunately, any and all possible acute infections in their breastfeeding baby or toddler have been wrongly given as a reason for mothers to stop or interrupt breastfeeding. The principles mentioned here also apply to any acute infant infection. It should be noted that in the young baby or toddler, many types of illness not caused by infection of the gastrointestinal tract may cause vomiting and diarrhea. Typical are infections such as, pneumonia or an infection of the urinary tract. Or, another example, appendicitis. If parents have any doubts that this is anything but a "tummy infection", the baby should be seen promptly by a doctor.

Gastroenteritis in the breastfed baby (vomiting and diarrhea due to infection)

Because of a whole system of interacting immune factors present in breastmilk, *exclusively* breastfed babies only rarely get gastroenteritis (an infection of the intestinal tract, usually due to a virus such as rotavirus, or less commonly, to bacteria or other microorganisms, such as giardia lamblia, a protozoa not rarely infecting children in day cares). If the exclusively breastfed baby does get gastroenteritis, it is unusual for it to be severe and almost always it is mild. And the best treatment for gastroenteritis is continued breastfeeding. The immune factors present in breastmilk not only help prevent gastroenteritis, *they also help to cure it*, and a number of factors present in breastmilk help the gut to heal.

Even partially breastfed babies/toddlers are relatively immune to getting gastroenteritis

Therefore, the first step in the treatment of gastroenteritis is **to continue breastfeeding**, as frequently as the baby desires. Not only will continued breastfeeding help in treating the infection, breastfeeding will maintain the baby's hydration. If the baby is already eating food but is not willing to eat

198

while sick, it is fine to stop other food temporarily and continue only with breastfeeding. On the other hand, if he is willing to eat food, he should be allowed to eat.

Usually, the only treatment that is necessary for the vast majority of cases of gastroenteritis is breastfeeding. According to the **World Health Organization**, page 10: "Breastfeeding should always be continued."

Breastfeeding is more than milk

It should not be forgotten how much comfort and security the baby or **toddler** receives from breastfeeding. This is particularly important when the baby is sick and perhaps feeling miserable.

Furthermore, a baby who will breastfeed when he is sick will give some reassurance to the parents that the baby is not so sick that they need to worry (more than parents usually worry). Thus, breastfeeding calms and reassures the baby; and the fact that the baby gets comfort from breastfeeding reassures and calms the mother.

But how do we deal with the vomiting and the diarrhea?

As long as the baby's hydration is well maintained by breastfeeding, there is no need for any other treatment. Just as most viral infections (colds, for example) will get better without "medical treatment" such as antibiotics, so will gastroenteritis, almost always.

The only other treatment that *might* be necessary, with a strong emphasis on "might", in more severe cases (rare in exclusively breastfed babies) is oral rehydration solution. Oral rehydration solutions of any kind are only necessary if breastfeeding is not keeping up with the baby's fluid requirements. However, some pediatricians or family physicians recommend special solutions "at the first sign of gastroenteritis", an absurd recommendation in the breastfed baby or toddler.

Breastfeeding alone may not keep up with the baby's fluid requirements, for example, if the mother's milk supply has decreased for whatever reason. In the usual situation, this would occur only once the baby is a toddler and is eating plenty of solids. However, once the baby wants to breastfeed more frequently, as is likely when the baby feels unwell, the milk supply will rise to the occasion. However, it is worth taking a look also at the article on **late onset decreased milk supply**.

On rare occasions, fluid loss in the baby/toddler is so rapid or abundant that the baby becomes lethargic and does not breastfeed. Oral rehydration fluids can be tried, but often if the baby or toddler refuses to breastfeed, the baby or toddler will not take oral rehydration fluids either. If this is the case, the parents should seek immediate medical care for the baby.

Oral rehydration fluids, inexpensive and easily available?

You might be interested that oral rehydrating solutions were developed for resource poor countries where the high cost of intravenous rehydration and the requirement for hospitalization to administer it put a great burden on health resources. Furthermore, in many resource poor places, the baby's hydration status and general well being are difficult to monitor when there are few health professionals for many sick babies or toddlers and the laboratory may not be as reliable as it should be. Oral rehydration solutions give the right amount of water and salts (sodium and potassium) for most babies and were especially made so that a litre (or quart, more or less) of the solution costs pennies. However, formula companies, always on the lookout for a quick and easy way of making money on sick babies, now sell oral rehydrating solutions (and maintenance solutions, which are unnecessary for the breastfed baby) for many dollars a litre. Last time I looked 1 litre of oral electrolyte solution was $12 (For a mixture of water and salt)! The profit margin must be huge.

Breastfeeding fits "doctor's orders"

In the past, before the formula companies got in on the game, diarrhea, especially if associated with vomiting, was treated with frequent, small amounts of fluid given to the baby. Flat soda pop (yuck) was a frequent recommendation. There was even an instruction by some doctors to alternate one cola (higher in sodium) with another (higher in potassium).

In fact, with breastfeeding, the baby gets frequent small feedings. The mother essentially keeps the baby at the breast, almost constantly. After the initial large intake of breastmilk at the beginning of a feeding (after the baby wakes up from a sleep, say), the baby will then be getting only small amounts of milk and the sucking at the breast helps the baby's stomach to empty (gastrocolic reflex), thus reducing vomiting. What if the baby vomits? The mother should put the baby back to the breast.

Even rarer in the exclusively breastfed baby is the need to rehydrate the baby with an intravenous solution.

Drugs to prevent vomiting and diarrhea

Medication to prevent vomiting and diarrhea is *almost* never necessary and usually does not work anyway. And these medicines can be harmful. Even if they do seem to work, it's not a good idea to use them. Vomiting and diarrhea are the body's method of ridding the gut of the virus or bacteria as well as the toxins formed by these germs. Vomiting and diarrhea in the presence of infection and toxins are a defence system! Treating the vomiting and diarrhea with medication may actually prolong the illness or cause it to recur.

• Dimenhydrinate (Gravol) is an antihistamine frequently used orally or as a rectal suppository to decrease vomiting. There is no good proof that it actually works to decrease vomiting. It can, however, cause excessive sleepiness (lethargy), which can confuse the clinical picture: Is the baby lethargic because of the drug or because he is becoming sicker? Such drugs should not be used especially for this very reason.

• Loperamide (Imodium) which is supposed to decrease the diarrhea should also not be used, for the same reason as mentioned above with regard to vomiting: diarrhea is the body's way of getting rid of the germs and toxins that cause the infection of the gut.

• Antibiotics are rarely if ever necessary in ordinary gastroenteritis since the majority of gastroenteritis is caused by viruses (norovirus or rotavirus, for example) and not bacteria. Even if caused by bacteria, antibiotics are not usually a good idea, except in unusual circumstances.

The best "drug" for vomiting and diarrhea due to infection is breastfeeding.

Prolonged diarrhea

In the typical case of gastroenteritis, the vomiting does not usually last for more than two or three days and the diarrhea rarely much longer than a week or so.

If the diarrhea lasts more than a week or so, it is often due to the fact that babies are eating low fat foods, typically and "traditionally" the "BRAT" diet widely recommended in the 1960s and before, as a slow "gentle" way to start food after gastroenteritis: the foods recommended were banana, rice, apple sauce and dry toast (hence BRAT). It has already been mentioned that if the child with gastroenteritis is willing to eat food, he should continue eating, but the food should not be low in fat. Adding fat to the child's diet will usually stop the "prolonged" diarrhea. In other words, get the child back on a normal diet. Note that breastmilk contains a lot of fat *especially* if **the mother has been breastfeeding for over a year**.

How can formula companies make even more money?

Various companies, including formula companies, have started to produce special products for diarrhea, especially "oral rehydrating solutions" with added carrots and rice. Really, carrots and rice? What for? All that stuff, being low in fat, will prolong the diarrhea and, of course bring in lots of money for the formula companies, who win three times over; once for the formula which put the child at risk for diarrhea, second for the "special" formulas for diarrhea, and third for this carrot and rice rubbish.

Why do pediatric societies not condemn their use?

Non-infectious diseases causing prolonged diarrhea

Breastfed babies or toddlers are not always spared such chronic diseases as coeliac disease, though they seem to have a lower risk than formula fed babies. If diarrhea is not resolving with increased intake of food after a few weeks, the child should be seen by the baby's doctor.

The bowel movements of the exclusively breastfed baby can seem to be diarrhea

The bowel movements of exclusively breastfed babies are often quite loose, even watery. Furthermore, they can be frequent (7 or 8 times or even more in a day is not rare) and can be green or seem to have no substance at all. **As long as the baby is drinking well at the breast**, is generally content, and gaining weight well, there is no problem. However, if not all of these three conditions apply, then something may be wrong. But note that a hungry baby who is sucking his fingers a lot of the time may seem a content baby, so this "sign" that all is okay is maybe not a good sign that all is okay.

One cause of frequent green bowel movements, sometimes even with small amounts of blood can be due to **late onset decreased milk supply**. The way to deal with this is to increase the baby's intake of milk from the breast.

Spitting up

Spitting up is different from vomiting in that vomiting is usually forceful and happens out of the ordinary pattern of the baby's behaviour. Often the baby is just not his "usual self".

With spitting up, the milk comes up often almost without anyone really noticing. Not the baby, and not the parents until the parent holding the baby feels his/her shoulder wet.

If **the baby is drinking well from the breast**, gaining weight well and is generally a happy baby, then spitting up, even a lot, is not bad. In fact, it is probably good. Breastmilk is full of immune factors (not just antibodies, but also dozens

203

of other immune factors as well that all interact with each other). These immune factors protect the baby from invasion by bacteria and viruses by lining the baby's mucous membranes (the linings of the gut, respiratory tract and elsewhere). This lining, this barrier, prevents the bacteria and viruses from entering the baby's body and blood. A baby who spits up has double protection, forming this barrier when the baby drinks the milk and it goes to the stomach and then when he spits it up. This may be particularly important as it is the upper part of the gut and respiratory tract which is most exposed to bacteria and viruses. We frequently use this example of how breastfeeding is so different from formula and bottle feeding. Spitting up formula, if all else is going well, is probably not bad. Spitting up breastmilk, if all else is going well, is probably good. Good, because the immune factors that cover the lining of the esophagus are replenished by spitting up.

BREASTFEEDING THE SICK BABY PART 2

When a baby is ill, either with an acute or a chronic illness, it is important to make every effort to protect the breastfeeding and to ensure that the mother continue breastfeeding him, if it is at all possible. And *it is almost always possible and desirable* to continue breastfeeding. In fact, it is not only possible, but it is also good for both the baby and the mother to continue breastfeeding. Sick babies need to continue breastfeeding, especially if the illness is due to an infection since the immune factors in breastmilk continue to be produced and even adapt to the bacteria or viruses which are making the baby ill. Since mothers and babies, being in such close physical contact, share bacteria and viruses, the mother will likely produce antibodies to the very infection that is causing the baby to be ill.

Furthermore, the baby is comforted by breastfeeding, especially when he is sick. Mothers also need to continue breastfeeding to prevent breast engorgement. More importantly, not only does breastfeeding comfort the baby but also, at the same time, **the mother is comforted by breastfeeding the baby.**

Are there some illnesses in the baby that absolutely require mothers to avoid breastfeeding?

There are very rare instances when a baby's illness requires interruption of breastfeeding or the baby not receiving breastmilk. Galactosemia, caused by a genetically transmitted inborn error of metabolism where the baby is unable to metabolize the sugar galactose properly is one such illness. Galactose is one of the two sugars making up lactose, the sugar present in breastmilk. The other sugar is glucose.

Because the baby cannot metabolise the galactose in the usual way, an alternate pathway of metabolism is taken which results in a toxic compound, galactitol, being formed. This toxic compound results in the baby developing liver disease, cataracts of the eye, brain injury and if removal of galactose from the baby's diet is not instituted, the baby will eventually die.

There is no way to remove galactose from breastmilk, at least at present, so a baby who has the full syndrome of galactosemia must not be breastfed. However, some babies have only "partial" galactosemia (Duarte variant) where they have some enzyme to metabolize galactose (as much as 10-25% of normal levels). These levels of enzyme result in the baby's being able to metabolize galactose adequately without suffering the devastating effects seen in classic galactosemia. They can and should breastfeed, just as any other baby. Babies with lower levels of enzyme can be partially breastfed. Incidentally, partial galactosemia is far more common than the full disease.

Other inborn errors of metabolism may also make breastfeeding more hazardous than artificial feeding. Tyrosinemia is, *perhaps*, one of them, but it is so rare that whether breastfeeding is possible for the baby has not been properly studied. The treatment of tyrosinemia is a "low protein diet", but breastmilk has significantly less protein than most formulas. Furthermore, since most of the protein in breastmilk is not absorbed from the baby's intestinal tract, it may be possible for a baby with tyrosinemia to be at least partially breastfed. (Lactoferrin and antibodies combined make up 60 to 70% of all the protein in breastmilk and are not absorbed at all by the baby).

As for maple syrup urine disease and many other extremely rare inborn errors of metabolism, we just don't know. The "default" treatments are usually special formulas, even though it may be possible for the babies to breastfeed. The idea in the minds of too many specialists is that since "formula is just like breastmilk" and ordinary formula is contraindicated in these rare diseases, therefore breastmilk and, obviously, breastfeeding are also thought to be contraindicated. Maybe they are, but assuming they are without proof, is just not good practice. Just as in the case of how much less protein is absorbed from the baby's gut, perhaps other differences between breastmilk and formula would make it possible for the baby to breastfeed, perhaps only partially, but safely.

Phenylketonuria (PKU)

Babies with phenylketonuria can breastfeed, at least partially.

Here is how, once upon a time, we helped babies with PKU to breastfeed at the Hospital for Sick Children in Toronto. "Once upon a time", because we understand that now, the mothers with babies with PKU are just simply told they can't breastfeed at all. But in those days the pediatrician in charge of the PKU clinic was supportive of breastfeeding. We think it is a pity that breastfeeding is not supported now, because the babies could breastfeed, and the babies would have not only breastmilk, but they would have that **special relationship of breastfeeding.** It is too bad however, that this notion of a close, physical and emotional relationship that is breastfeeding does not fit the "medical model".

The issue is that babies with PKU cannot metabolize the amino acid phenylalanine to another amino acid tyrosine, and the buildup of phenylalanine results in brain damage and cataracts amongst other things. However, phenylalanine is an *essential* amino acid, meaning that you need it for proper metabolism. So, the baby with PKU needs phenylalanine, *but not too much.*

Back in the 1980s, when we had just started the breastfeeding clinic at the Hospital for Sick Children in Toronto, the people from the phenylketonuria clinic came to me and asked how they could help mothers breastfeed longer. The babies were stopping breastfeeding very soon after birth, usually by the time the baby was 2 or 3 weeks old. And it's easy to see why.

Before our suggestions on how to help the mothers breastfeed, the mothers were told to feed in this way:

1. The baby would be weighed before the feeding.

2. The mother would then feed the baby 10 minutes on each side (by the clock).

3. The mother would weigh the baby after the feeding at the breast.

4. The mother would give the rest of the feeding (calculated by the dietician to make sure the baby didn't get too much phenylalanine) as low phenylalanine formula.

207

One needs only a smidgen of breastfeeding knowledge to know why this would not work.

1. The mother had to carry the scale with her wherever she went. Not very practical, and what if she forgot the scale?

2. One can easily imagine that the mother would be anxious about the baby getting "too much breastmilk" and thus causing the baby to get too much phenylalanine resulting, likely, in the mother restricting the baby's time on the breast.

3. The babies started to prefer the bottle, which is not surprising.

We came up with this solution

1. The dietitian would calculate the approximate quantity of low phenylalanine formula the baby would require.

2. The mother would give this amount of low phenylalanine formula at the beginning of the feeding with a **lactation aid at the breast**.

3. Then, allow the baby to finish the feeding on the breast without timing the feeding.

4. The amount of low phenylalanine formula would be adjusted depending on the blood levels of phenylalanine that were normally followed anyway, regardless of feeding method.

   We learned that the low phenylalanine formula was thicker than usual formulas, so it did not pass easily through the usual 5 French tube we used for **supplementing at the breast**. So, we used a larger 8 French tube which has a wider bore through which the milk will pass. And it worked well.

   What happened? During the first year, breastfeeding continued much longer.

1. One baby breastfed to 18 months of age

2. Several breastfed to 6 months

3. One baby who had atypical PKU was able to be breastfed exclusively for six months

Premature babies and babies with congenital heart disease and other illnesses

It is uncommon for premature babies in North America to leave hospital breastfeeding exclusively. One reason is that few special care units practice true **Kangaroo Mother Care**. In addition, mothers are often told that **premature babies cannot breastfeed until they are 34 weeks gestation, which is incorrect.** Experience from Scandinavia shows that some premature babies can start going to the breast by 27 weeks gestation.

Furthermore, the lack of confidence that many neonatologists have in breastmilk and breastfeeding results in too many babies getting "fortifiers" mixed in with breastmilk (the quotation marks are to suggest that when "fortifiers" are used unnecessarily, as they often are, they should be called breastmilk "weakeners"). "Fortifiers" are mixed with expressed breastmilk to increase nutrients that are felt to be missing or in inadequate amounts in breastmilk alone. **The use of "fortifiers"** may sometimes be necessary, but not routinely, as is usual in many special care units.

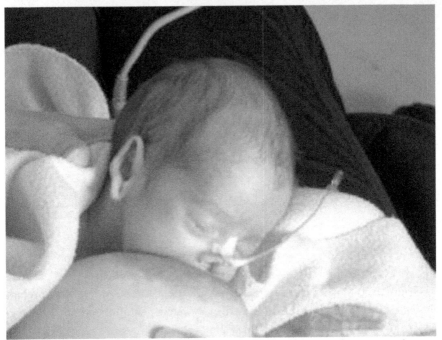

This baby is 2 weeks old. He was born at 28 weeks gestation. He is latched on and drinking from the breast.

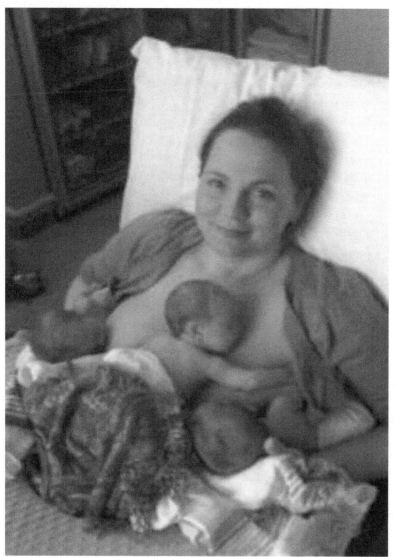

Triplets born prematurely managed to get out of the NICU without ever getting *bottles or having "fortifier" added to the breastmilk.*

Babies with congenital heart malformations, cardiomyopathy and other heart problems

Is it important for these babies to breastfeed? Of course! Babies with heart diseases need **comfort and security** just like all babies, maybe even more, as they are frequently subjected to painful tests and treatments. Furthermore, they need the immunity provided by breastfeeding because they are often in hospital for long periods of time and we know that hospitals are not the best places to avoid infections. Infection in a baby with congenital heart disease can be fatal.

These babies are often fed by bottles because it is thought, *wrongly*, that breastfeeding is too tiring for a baby with heart disease.

The idea that breastfeeding is tiring for the baby arises from the mistaken belief that "babies transfer milk", in other words that babies "suck milk out of the breast" and that this is "hard work" for the baby which results in the baby using a lot of calories. But this is not understanding breastfeeding and how breastfeeding works. Babies do not "suck milk out of the breast". Babies stimulate milk to be released from the breast, and **the mother "transfers" the milk to the baby**.

The other issue that arises with babies with congenital heart malformations is that some of them have heart failure. Thus, cardiologists limit the amount of liquid (including breastmilk) that the baby can receive. I would think that careful physical examination and close monitoring of these babies will allow the babies to breastfeed without limiting the frequency or the length of time the baby is at the breast.

If it becomes truly necessary to limit the amount of breastmilk the baby receives, it is reasonable, given the importance of breastfeeding (**breastfeeding is more than the milk**) to increase the diuretics ("water pills"), which cause the baby to lose fluid and other medications that stimulate the heart to work more efficiently or decrease the work of the heart. True, higher doses of medication may cause more side effects, but we believe strongly that breastfeeding is worth the risk, especially when babies are sick.

It is also possible to keep intravenous fluids to a minimum.

And if it is truly necessary to limit the amount of breastmilk a baby gets. The mother can express her milk just before a feeding and give back the baby the "required" amount of milk with the **lactation aid** at the "dry" breast.

Chylothorax

A special situation arises when a baby develops a chylothorax. This problem usually arises after cardiac surgery, but an occasional baby is born with it for no obvious reason. In the case of chylothorax after heart surgery, the thoracic duct, which brings lymph back to the heart to be returned to the blood is unavoidably nicked. This results with lymph accumulating in the space between the lung and the chest wall.

A chylothorax is usually treated with a low-fat diet and chest drainage. The reason for the low-fat diet is that it decreases the lymph flow in the thoracic duct. A low fat diet is fine for an adult who can manage for a while on a low-fat diet, but not for a baby, who needs fat to grow and develop.

The chest drainage is done as it would be for an adult or older child, but usually the cardiologists insist that the baby must not breastfeed but must drink a "special" formula with medium chain triglycerides, instead of breastmilk and other formulas which contain significant amounts of long chain triglycerides. Why medium chain triglycerides? Interestingly they do not get absorbed into the lymph like long chain triglycerides, but instead, are absorbed directly into the blood, so do not increase lymph flow.

But something can be done. Instead of special formula, the mother's breastmilk can be used instead. The milk is centrifuged, and the fat which is at the top of the centrifuged milk is taken off and stored for later use. The people in the nutrition department then add medium chain triglycerides to the milk. It's not quite breastmilk but it's better than the formula.

Just before feeding the baby, the mother pumps out as much milk as practical, and feeds the baby breastmilk with the medium chain triglycerides prepared by the nutrition department with a **lactation aid at the breast** on the "dry breast" (recently pumped breast). The baby will probably still get some breastmilk from

213

the breast, but the formula with medium chain triglycerides is not completely free of long and short chain triglycerides either. Using the lactation aid on the "dry" breast will prevent the problem of the baby refusing to latch on to the breast after several weeks, which the treatment of chylothorax may require.

The baby with cystic fibrosis

Is it important for these babies to breastfeed? Of course! Babies with cystic fibrosis need **comfort and security** just like all babies, maybe even more, as they are frequently subjected to painful tests and treatments. Furthermore, they need the immunity provided by breastfeeding because they are often in hospital for long periods of time and we know that hospitals are not the best places to avoid infections. Infection in a baby with cystic fibrosis can be fatal.

Most babies with cystic fibrosis have difficulty digesting their food, probably also including breastmilk. But breastmilk does contain lipase (the enzyme that digests fat), proteases (the enzymes that digest protein) and amylase (which breaks down complex carbohydrate). It is likely that unless the baby has a relatively mild form of pancreatic enzyme insufficiency, the baby will still need extra enzymes, but maybe smaller amounts.

The enzymes can be given to the baby by an open glass cup.

The baby/toddler with type 1 diabetes

Breastfed babies can develop type 1 diabetes, though uncommonly. It was thought that in the 1990s that exclusively breastfed babies had a much lower rate because they were not exposed to cow milk protein. They were not completely protected because, as with many diseases, development of the disease is caused by more than one factor, often several factors acting together. In the case of type 1 diabetes, there is more to it than just avoiding cow milk protein. A baby may develop diabetes when the baby has the genetic background that puts him or her at risk, *plus* an infection with a virus at a critical moment. It is likely that breastfeeding protects, perhaps by decreasing the risk of the infection, but the protection is not complete.

214

The results of a recently published **study** that has been going on since the mid 1990s has shown that you cannot decrease the risk of the baby developing diabetes by avoiding cow milk protein early in life. The study looked at babies who were mostly started on breastfeeding but weaned either to a cow milk based formula or a hydrolyzed formula. At first there was no group of exclusive breastfeeding babies to the recommended 6 months, and the average age of adding formula was 2.5 months. Essentially, this was a study that did not disprove that breastfeeding protected, because exclusive breastfeeding was rare in the study groups.

Should breastfeeding be stopped when a baby/toddler develops diabetes type 1?

When a baby or toddler does develop type 1 diabetes, the pediatric endocrinologists usually will recommend that breastfeeding be stopped. The apparent reason for this is that they want to carefully control the diet, making sure the child gets a certain amount of protein, fat and carbohydrate.

But it is often very difficult for the mother to stop breastfeeding, especially a **toddler**. And there are many reasons to continue breastfeeding. It *might* be a little more difficult to control the blood sugar levels if the child is breastfeeding, but the **comfort and security** the child gets while breastfeeding are important and more than outweigh the problem with somewhat higher blood sugars. In fact, when we were training we were taught that we should keep a young baby or toddler's blood sugar levels a little high, to prevent the baby from developing too low blood sugars which are more of a risk for the child than somewhat higher blood sugars for the few years the baby may be breastfed.

With computer technology now available in the form of special pens that send information to cell phones and that can get all sorts of information on the state of the baby's blood sugar, how many carbohydrates he's taking in and several other pieces of information that help regulate the blood sugar as best possible. Even less reason to stop breastfeeding than a few years ago.

It is impossible to discuss every possible illness a baby or toddler may have, but with an understanding (health worker's and mother's) of how breastfeeding works, with a commitment to breastfeeding, with good support, good hands on help, and with some imagination and creativity, breastfeeding, and not just "breastmilk", can not only be salvaged but actually made to work very well despite many types of illness too frequent and varied to discuss here. These examples can give an approach which may work for other illnesses that babies or toddlers may be born with or develop.

Why bother with all this?

Because breastmilk and even more importantly, *breastfeeding* are important to the physical and emotional health of the baby as well as of the mother's. Especially the baby who is sick, who needs the physical and emotional contact of breastfeeding even more than a healthy baby, who also needs it. And the mother needs breastfeeding also because she gets the physical and emotional contact of breastfeeding. And she will feel that she is contributing to the treatment of her baby. And she will be right. Too bad that only a few pediatricians, neonatologists and other health professionals seem to understand this.

BREASTFEEDING AND MATERNAL ILLNESS PART 1

Mothers are frequently told they must stop breastfeeding if they are sick, both for acute and chronic illness. In fact, it almost seems as if maternal illness is taken as an opportunity to "give mothers permission to stop breastfeeding" instead of re-assuring them that they can safely continue breastfeeding. Some health professionals, I hope very few, have stated that since "breastfeeding is such a burden on the mother, that if she is ill, it is best not to continue breastfeeding".

We should note here that if we helped mothers as we should with establishing and continuing breastfeeding, breastfeeding would *not* be a burden, but rather, easy, relaxing, and enjoyable. Not only can the mother safely continue breastfeeding, but continuing breastfeeding is good physically and emotionally for both for the mother and the baby.

The issue of **maternal medication and breastfeeding** has been addressed in another chapter as has the question of **acute illness in the breastfed baby** and **chronic illness in the breastfed baby.**

Illness sometimes requires drug treatment and breastfeeding mothers are frequently being told they must stop breastfeeding for the **medication** they may have to take. However, in the vast majority of cases, this advice is inappropriate and clearly incorrect. Sometimes mothers are told to stop for what can only be called bizarre reasons. For example, a mother who was breastfeeding a 6 month old and had a recent flare-up of her Crohn's disease was told that the flare-up was due to prolactin and that she would need to stop breastfeeding. I guess prolactin works really slowly because prolactin was being secreted in large quantities during the pregnancy and was important in the making of breastmilk from immediately after birth. It seems that breastfeeding can be blamed for making every illness worse. Sometimes it seems that for some doctors, any reason is good enough to tell mothers to stop breastfeeding.

It should be noted that the symptoms of many chronic diseases, especially, it seems, inflammatory diseases improve during pregnancy. Thus, it may seem to many observers that somehow breastfeeding is responsible for flare-ups or relapses of symptoms. As well, some chronic illnesses get worse during breastfeeding because mothers stop taking their medications, having been told they cannot take them while breastfeeding.

Breastfeeding protects the baby when the mother has a contagious illness

Most infectious diseases, whether they are due to a bacterium or a virus, are usually *most* contagious *before* the person with the infection has any symptoms of illness or the person even knows having been exposed to an infection. Thus, the breastfeeding baby is exposed to the bacterium or the virus for days, even weeks in the case of some infections, before the mother feels sick or has fever or even knows she has been in contact with an infectious disease.

It is true that most viruses have what is called a "viremic" stage, when the virus is present in the blood and thus, theoretically, could appear in the milk, but this stage occurs soon after the mother has been infected and usually lasts only a few hours. The viremic stage occurs, generally, before the mother knows she has been infected. Therefore, stopping breastfeeding at a time when the mother is already obviously sick implies stopping when the baby needs the protection of breastfeeding the most.

It is remarkable that so many health professionals do not seem to understand this. Was the mother not exposed and infected before she consulted the physician? Was the baby not breastfeeding during that time?

It's not just about antibodies

Almost everyone seems to know that breastmilk contains antibodies and think they know how the antibodies protect the baby. But when it comes down to the crunch, it seems that nobody really believes the antibodies make any difference. But those antibodies *do* matter, they *do* protect. There are, normally, antibodies in the milk, even if the mother is not sick. But when a mother is exposed to an infection, new antibodies specifically directed against the infection to which she was exposed, begin to be produced.

How does this work? See the drawings below from an article that was published in **Scientific American** in 1995. When a mother is exposed to a bacterium or virus, the bacterium or virus come into contact with special cells called M cells in her intestinal wall. Unlike other cells in the mother's intestines, these do not try to reject the microbe, but actually, deliberately, if we can say a cell has free will, absorb the bacterium or virus.

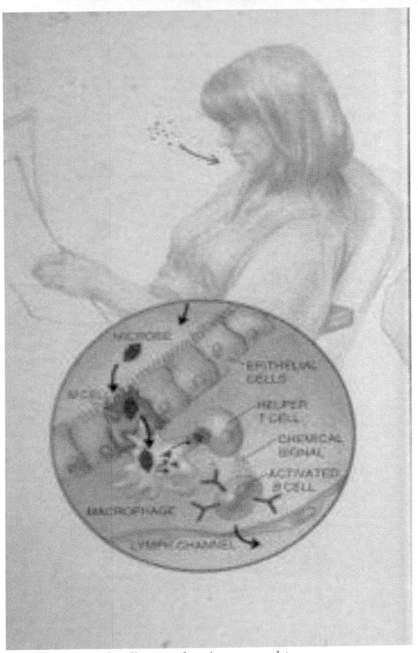

When a breastfeeding mother is exposed to a
microbe (virus or bacterium), her body starts making
antibodies to the microbe. These antibodies will soon appear
in the milk to protect the baby.

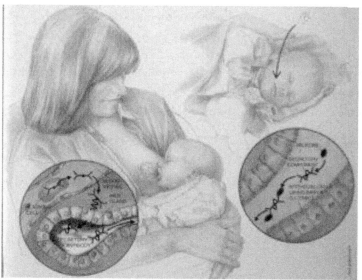

The infectious agent to which the mother has been exposed has stimulated the production of antibodies to the infectious agent. These antibodies now enter the milk and help to protect the baby.

In the intestine, just below the layer exposed to intestinal fluid, information about the microbe (virus or bacterium or fungus) passes through a number of cells normally found under the intestinal wall and one sort, called a B lymphocyte, is changed by exposure to that information. This B lymphocyte enters the lymph and soon, usually within about 24 hours, has now become a plasma cell (lower photo) and is producing antibodies to the very microbe to which the mother has been exposed not that long ago. These antibodies enter the milk and help to protect the baby against the infectious agent to which the mother was exposed. Note that this all is usually occurring even before the mother knows she is sick. But note also that it is the exposure to the microbe that sets all this in motion. The mother does not actually have to become ill for all this to happen. We are all exposed to infections from time to time, but we don't necessarily become ill because of the exposure.

In the meantime, breastmilk is providing the baby with many other immune substances (lactoferrin, lysozyme to mention only 2 of many) which help the baby fight off any microbe to which he was exposed. And the antibodies and other substances form a barrier along the mucous membranes (the internal linings) of the baby's body which protect the baby by preventing the microbes from entering his body (the inside of the gastrointestinal tract is considered outside the body). This barrier prevents bacteria and viruses from entering into the baby's body and is an important way the antibodies and other immune factors present in breastmilk protect the baby against infectious agents.

Unfortunately, not a rare approach

If it weren't so sad, it would be comical to imagine this not rare scenario (a true story, incidentally): A mother develops an upper respiratory infection (a cold). She is seen by the family doctor and is told she cannot breastfeed because 1. The baby will catch the cold from the milk and 2. The mother needs to start on amoxicillin (a very commonly used antibiotic) and the baby will get the antibiotic in the milk. The question of why it would have been necessary to see a physician for a cold is another issue which we will leave at this point and the question of antibiotics (also unnecessary for a cold) **getting into the milk** has been discussed in a previous chapter.

But what about the virus that caused the mother's cold? To begin with, mothers and babies, especially breastfeeding mothers, are in close contact much of the time, so whoever gave the mother the virus probably also gave it to the baby as well. But even if not, the mother had the cold virus for a couple of days before she felt ill, so the baby has been receiving immune factors from the breastmilk, including those new antibodies.

Furthermore, breastfeeding, the act of breastfeeding, *beyond breastmilk*, also protects the baby. The very act of breastfeeding decreases stress, decreases cortisol levels in the baby, decreases crying (and thus stress) and the physical contact, the skin to skin contact during breastfeeding has been shown to improve the immune response of the baby and lowers the inflammatory response in the baby which is what frequently causes the damage that occurs during infections.

To end the story, the mother contacted us a few days after the first visit to the doctor. She had visited the doctor a second time and called us immediately after the second visit. I will always remember how she said: "There is something I don't understand. Today I went to the doctor again because my baby started a cold. The doctor put him on amoxicillin. There is something I don't understand."

Well, of course, the whole episode makes no sense at all. To begin with, the mother should have been advised to continue breastfeeding. And she should not have been put on an antibiotic. If she had continued breastfeeding, it is unlikely that the baby would have developed the cold. Okay, he might have. But chances are the cold would have been milder.

After all is said and done?

1. The mother went to the doctor for a cold, received incorrect advice about breastfeeding her baby and received a prescription for an antibiotic that was useless for her problem and could have significant side effects.

2. The mother would likely have had to express her milk, which is a nuisance.

3. The baby might have rejected the breast after two days of bottle feeding.

4. The baby's **microbiome** (gut flora) were likely changed significantly by exposure to an antibiotic and being fed formula for two day.

All for no reason!

BREASTFEEDING AND MATERNAL ILLNESS PART 2

See also **Breastfeeding and Maternal Illness Part 1**

Some infectious diseases

A full discussion of all infectious diseases that could affect the mother and breastfeeding could result in a book the size of War and Peace, so we will try to deal, briefly, only with those that seem to cause the most problems for doctors and, as a result, for the breastfeeding mothers. It should be assumed that if an infectious disease is not included here, that it is safe and preferable for mothers to continue breastfeeding.

Hepatitis

Hepatitis is an infection of the liver and of most concern with regard to breastfeeding are hepatitis A, B and C. There are other hepatitis viruses, maybe named up to hepatitis Z by now, but they are uncommon causes of liver infection.

Hepatitis A

This virus is typical of viruses as already mentioned in **Breastfeeding and Maternal Illness Part 1** in the sense that by the time the mother is aware she is unwell, the viremic phase has already passed for many days or even weeks (the viremic phase is when the virus is found in the blood). Though infection of others is very possible from virus in the bowel movements, infection from bowel movements is no longer likely either. Once the mother has symptoms, the virus is no longer in the intestinal tract. In other words, by the time the mother is obviously sick, she can no longer pass the infection to the baby, not by being with the baby or by breastfeeding.

If, at some earlier moment, the baby did pick up the virus, breastfeeding will help decrease the risk of his becoming ill even if he becomes infected. If he does get infected while the mother still has no symptoms but is infectious, continued breastfeeding will likely diminish the severity of the infection even if the baby or toddler does become ill. Note that being infected does not mean becoming sick.

It is true that hepatitis, if severe (it can be mild or even asymptomatic), can cause the mother to be extremely tired, with abdominal pain (due to the stretching of the lining of the liver) and to having no appetite, as well as feeling weak. All this may make it difficult for her to care for the baby. It is best that the mother go to bed with the baby and nurse him in bed. It would also be best if she not be responsible for other requirements of the baby or other chores and working outside the home during this time.

Hepatitis B

Hepatitis B is similar to hepatitis A in that the symptoms are very similar; jaundice, fatigue, abdominal pain. As with hepatitis A, not everyone who is infected develops the illness. However, unlike hepatitis A, about 10 to 15% of all people who are infected with hepatitis B become chronic carriers of the virus and this is possible even if they did not develop an acute hepatitis B illness. This means their bodily fluids may be infectious even though they have no symptoms of the disease. However, like hepatitis A, by the time the mother develops symptoms, it is possible the virus already passed on to the baby. There is no evidence though, that the virus will enter the milk once the mother has symptoms or during the carrier state. In any case, breastfeeding can still protect the baby.

In some jurisdictions, it is recommended that all babies receive hepatitis B vaccine at birth. In other jurisdictions, it is strongly recommended that the newborns of mothers who are chronic carriers of the hepatitis B, get the hepatitis B vaccine.

Hepatitis C

The clinical picture of hepatitis C is similar to hepatitis A and hepatitis B, though it is frequently milder and very often asymptomatic. As with hepatitis B, however, a chronic carrier state is not rare with hepatitis C.

There is **no evidence that breastfeeding can transmit the infection to the baby**.

Drug treatment of the carrier state of hepatitis C is now available.

Human Immunodeficiency Virus (HIV)

This is a very special virus in the sense that it attacks and destroys the immune system. Most infections so far known to medicine do not do that. Furthermore, it can be transferred to the baby in breastmilk. Thus, until recently, breastfeeding was considered contraindicated where formula feeding was considered safe and feasible (which it is not in many resource-poor areas).

Now, however, with effective medication that will treat the mother and also the baby, there has been a change in the recommendations for breastfeeding. When drug treatment of an HIV positive pregnant woman is begun during the pregnancy and the baby is started on treatment immediately after birth, breastfeeding has become possible and again preferable for both the mother and baby. The World Health Organization has published this **statement**, that when the mother and baby are treated, breastfeeding should be encouraged.

Herpes Viruses

At present, there are 9 different herpes viruses known to cause disease in humans. It is likely that in the future more will be discovered. In addition to sores on skin, lips, mouth, genitals, and conjunctivae of the eyes, herpes viruses also cause chicken pox, infectious mononucleosis, and herpes zoster (shingles). It should be noted that the vast majority of infections with herpes viruses do not cause symptoms. The person is infected but does not develop disease as is true of many types of infections.

Herpes virus 1 and 2

These two viruses can cause infectious lesions of the lips and mouth (herpes 1) and genitals (herpes 2, occasionally herpes 1).

The most common situation we run across occurs when a breastfeeding toddler, usually, develops herpes stomatitis, ulcers in the mouth, that are painful enough sometimes to prevent the child from breastfeeding or eating or drinking anything at all. Usually, though the child may refuse food and liquids, he will continue to breastfeed and should be encouraged to do so. However, refusal of *all* liquids and food including breastfeeding, occasionally requires the child to be admitted to hospital for intravenous fluids to maintain hydration. We believe that if the child continues with breastfeeding, hospitalization is rarely, if ever, needed. But if the child is admitted to the hospital, he should continue to breastfeed as soon as he will accept the breast.

Sometimes, the breastfeeding mother develops sores on her nipples which can be very painful. As with the other infections discussed previously, the incubation period of herpes virus before the toddler develops the sores is about a week, so the mother will have been infected by the breastfeeding child several days before the child had sores. The following photo shows herpes virus infection of the nipples transmitted from the baby.

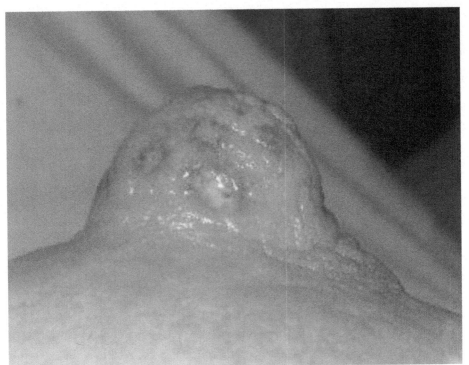

Nipple of a mother whose toddler developed herpetic stomatitis (infection in the mouth) about 3 or 4 days before she developed these painful sores. She continued breastfeeding through the pain and in about 1 week, the sores were healing and pain was gone.

It is best if the mother continues to breastfeed if she can. Hand expressing her milk and feeding it to the baby, preferably with an open cup rather than a bottle, is better than pumping because proper hand expression does not including squeezing the nipples. The milk can be fed to the baby by open cup or spoon, or mixed with solids, if the baby/toddler will take anything by mouth. A pump can cause pain of the nipple and frequently does.

Lyme Disease

Lyme disease is caused by a bacterium which is transmitted from the bite of a tick (actually, there are several different bacteria that can cause Lyme disease in different parts of North America and the rest of the world). It is a disease which can affect several systems in the body, including the skin, the joints, the heart and the central nervous system. Facial nerve paralysis, though it can have several causes, should make the physician think of the possibility of Lyme disease. It is generally believed that the tick needs to be attached for many hours before the bacterium of Lyme disease can infect the bitten person, though not everyone agrees with this.

Living Lyme disease bacteria have never been found in breastmilk, though one study has found DNA of the bacterium in the breastmilk. DNA, however does not transmit the infection.

However, even if the bacterium did pass into the milk, it is extremely unlikely that the bacterium would pass the **barrier of immune factors that prevent most viruses and bacteria from getting through to the intestinal wall and entering into the baby's blood stream**. The bacterium needs to get past that barrier, and then penetrate the intestinal wall to get into the bloodstream of the baby to cause infection. Thus, the likelihood of transmitting the virus to the baby by breastfeeding and causing infection in the baby are extremely low, approaching zero.

The question of whether the drug of choice for treatment of Lyme disease in the mother, doxycycline, is contraindicated during breastfeeding comes up frequently. **It is not contraindicated during breastfeeding**, though some experts recommend limiting treatment to 3 to 6 weeks. Treatment of Lyme disease does not usually require treatment with doxycycline for as long as 6 weeks.

Influenza A and B

Every winter there is an epidemic of influenza across the world, some years influenza being much more severe than in other years. People start falling ill in the fall and often the epidemic continues into the spring. The influenza viruses are not, essentially different from other infections from the point of view of breastfeeding. The mother often does not know she has been exposed and should she be infected with one of the viruses, she may not develop the illness. Even if she falls ill, she will have been infectious to her baby or toddler for a few days before she knows she is ill. Thus, the baby has usually been exposed to the virus before the mother knows any of the above.

It is best, when the mother has influenza, to continue breastfeeding, just as it is best with all acute infections.

Some non-infectious diseases

There is a host of **inflammatory and autoimmune diseases** such as rheumatoid arthritis, lupus erythematosus, idiopathic thrombocytopenic purpura, autoimmune hemolytic anemia, autoimmune thyroiditis (Hashimoto thyroiditis, for example), and many more, which are associated with and probably caused by antibodies against various tissues of the body. In the case of rheumatoid arthritis, it is to the joints of the body; in lupus erythematosus to several different tissues of the body; in idiopathic thrombocytopenic purpura to the platelets in the blood which help stop bleeding, to the thyroid gland in autoimmune thyroiditis, and so on.

Can't breastfeed because of antibodies in the milk?

Many physicians seem to believe that the mother cannot breastfeed because the antibodies causing the diseases may enter the milk and cause the disease in the baby. This is patently false.

Frequently, the reason for telling mothers not to breastfeed is the **medication** the mothers must take not only for the illnesses below, but also medications prescribed for multiple sclerosis (probably the illness we get asked about most), and postpartum depression. As mentioned in a **another chapter**, the vast majority of drugs do not require a mother to stop breastfeeding.

Many mothers who have conditions caused by antibodies against their own tissues (Graves' disease, Hashimoto thyroiditis, lupus erythematosus, idiopathic thrombocytopenic purpura, autoimmune hemolytic anemia, rheumatoid arthritis and others) are told that they should not breastfeed because the antibodies causing their disease will get into the milk and cause the same disease in the baby.

This is simply not true. First of all, the sIgA, which is the main antibody in breastmilk, making up at least 95% of all the antibodies in the milk, does not get absorbed from the baby's gut, so it cannot get into the baby's body and cause disease. Secondly, the antibodies that cause these diseases such as rheumatoid arthritis are not of the IgA type and, in any case, they would not get into the milk in any but insignificant amounts. Even if they did, they would be destroyed in the baby's stomach (sIgA does not get destroyed because it has that J chain which protects it from digestive enzymes). And even if the antibodies causing autoimmune diseases somehow did get past the digestive enzymes, they also would not be absorbed into the baby's body.

So, if the mother has a condition in which antibodies in her body attack her own tissues, the mother can and should breastfeed her baby with confidence that she is doing the best for her baby and not worry about the antibodies getting into the milk and causing a problem for the baby. And if she is taking **medication** for this condition, she should also continue breastfeeding.

But the baby could be born with the same problem!

True, in conditions such as those mentioned above caused by the mother producing antibodies to her own tissues, the baby is often born with the same problems as the mother. But that is because the antibodies get to the baby during the pregnancy, not from breastmilk.

Idiopathic thrombocytopenic purpura

A baby whose mother has idiopathic thrombocytopenia purpura (where the mother has low platelets caused by antibodies against platelets, thus causing them to be destroyed, and making it possible to bleed excessively) will often be born with low platelets as well, since the mother's antibodies passed *through the placenta* to the baby during the pregnancy, but **not from the breastmilk**. This effect on the baby is obvious because the platelet count is easy to

231

measure, a routine part of the blood count along with hemoglobin, hematocrit and white blood cell counts.

The baby's low platelet count can be present for a few weeks after birth, but only rarely is the platelet count so low as to cause a real risk of bleeding. With time, usually by six or eight weeks after the baby's birth, the platelet count of the baby will be rising since the antibodies will be disappearing from his blood.

Autoimmune hemolytic anemia

Another situation in which the problem is easy to measure occurs when the mother has autoimmune hemolytic anemia, a condition due to antibodies against her red blood cells, resulting in anemia. The baby can be born with his red blood cell count low because of the antibodies that passed into his body *during the pregnancy*. Both idiopathic thrombocytopenic purpura and autoimmune hemolytic anemia almost always improve without specific treatment unless the baby's platelets, in the one case, or the red blood cells, in the other, are very low and require transfusion, which is only rarely necessary.

Hyperthyroidism, Graves' Disease, Hashimoto's thyroiditis

Yet another situation occurs when the mother has Graves' disease which causes hyperthyroidism (overactive thyroid). The antibodies in the mother's blood *cross the placenta*, as with the other conditions discussed above and the baby is born with signs of hyperthyroidism; rapid heart rate (over 160/minute), jitteriness, high blood pressure and even congestive heart failure if severe. Poor weight gain may also occur. Treatment of the baby's symptoms is possible with drugs that block the effect of the overactive thyroid. But again, there is no reason to restrict breastfeeding.

In *rare* cases, however, the baby continues to have the above problems much longer than the usual 6 to 8 weeks. It seems very *unlikely* that this is due to the continued presence of antibodies from the pregnancy which disappear from the baby's blood within the first few weeks at most, and as mentioned above, impossible to explain as being due to antibodies in the milk. More likely, there are cytokines, small proteins that can affect immune responsiveness in the baby and result in continued problems.

A prolonged effect on the blood cells or platelets as well as other such syndromes, longer, say, than two to three months is unusual, even rare, and no reason to tell the mother not to breastfeed from birth as is often done. Should prolonged low platelets or low hemoglobin or other syndromes occur, longer than 3 or 4 months, despite treatment such as transfusion or oral corticosteroids in the baby, stopping breastfeeding may be considered. It should be pointed out that low platelets, unless severe, are not usually associated with a high risk of bleeding.

BREASTFEEDING THE PREMATURE: PART 1

If mothers and full-term babies generally do not get good help with the initiation of breastfeeding in most hospitals, and they don't, mothers and *premature* babies get even less help and more undermining of breastfeeding.

Premature babies need to be in incubators?

The assumption that has become a hard and fast rule, that premature babies need to be in incubators is simply not true in most cases. Premature babies (and full-term babies) in **Kangaroo Mother Care** (skin to skin contact for much of the day) are happier and with regard to their physiologic and metabolic functions **stabilize sooner after birth**. And they are more stable even *after* the first hours after birth. They are **generally more stable** from the point of view of heart rate, **respiratory rate**, blood pressure, blood sugar than babies in incubators. Premature babies in KMC (Kangaroo Mother Care) are less likely to stop breathing for prolonged periods of time (more than 20 seconds is considered prolonged) or develop bradycardias (slow heart rate) when in skin to skin contact with the parents. They maintain their **skin temperature** better as well. Keeping the premature baby's temperature in the normal and stable was the premise of keeping them in incubators in the first place, but skin to skin care does it better.

Furthermore, **studies** show that skin-to-skin care of mothers with their babies during venipuncture (blood letting) had a pain-relieving effect. And, very importantly, they are more likely to **begin breastfeeding earlier to leave hospital breastfeeding and breastfeeding** *exclusively* when the mother and baby have been in Kangaroo Mother Care.

Although this information has been known and readily available and published in peer-reviewed medical journals since the early 1980s at least, it seems that in most NICUs around the world, Kangaroo Mother Care is simply not done.

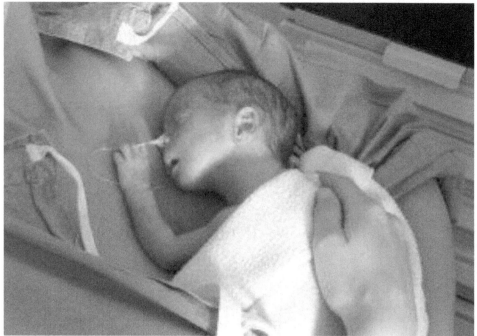

Premature baby, born at 28 weeks gestation, now 1 week old in skin to skin contact with his mother. Kangaroo Mother Care helps the baby maintain his body heat, heart rate, respiratory rate, blood sugar level, blood pressure and encourages early initiation of breastfeeding.

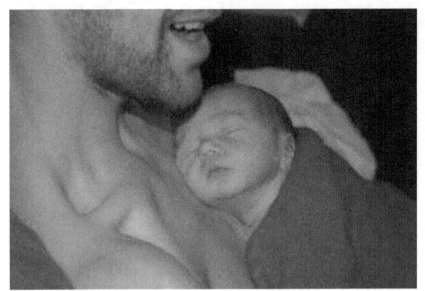

Fathers can also do skin to skin care with their baby. Kangaroo father care?

Here are *just a few* of the many articles showing the positive results of Kangaroo Mother Care for premature babies. There are many **more studies if you need them,** but a complete list could go to hundreds of studies that are available in the scientific literature.

Föhe K, Kropf S, Avenarius S. **Skin-to-Skin Contact Improves Gas Exchange in Premature Infants.** *Journal of Perinatology* 2000;5:311315.

"During skin-to-skin contact, preterm infants not only remain clinically stable but also show a more efficient gas exchange. Although the patient is removed (transferred) from the incubator, there is no risk of hypothermia even in infants of <1000 gm."

Charpak N, Ruiz-Peláez JG, Figueroa de C Z, Charpak Y. **A Randomized, Controlled Trial of Kangaroo Mother Care: Results of Follow-Up at 1 Year of Corrected Age.** *Pediatrics* 2001;108:1072-1079

"These results support earlier findings of the beneficial effects of KMC on mortality and growth. Use of this technique would humanize the practice of neonatology, promote breastfeeding, and shorten the neonatal hospital stay without compromising survival, growth, or development."

Bergman NJ, Linley LL, Fawcus SR. **Randomized controlled trial of skin-to-skin contact from birth versus conventional incubator for physiological stabilization in 1200- to 2199-gram newborns.** Acta Pædiatr 2004;93:779-785

"Newborn care provided by skin-to-skin contact on the mother's chest results in better physiological outcomes and stability than the same care provided in closed servo-controlled incubators. The cardio-respiratory instability seen in separated infants in the first 6 h is consistent with mammalian "protest-despair" biology, and with "hyper-arousal and dissociation" response patterns described in human infants: newborns should not be separated from their mothers."

Nyqvist KH, Anderson GC, Bergman N *et al.* **Towards universal Kangaroo Mother Care: recommendations and report from the First European conference and Seventh International Workshop on Kangaroo Mother Care.** Acta Pædiatrica 2010;99:820-*826*

"Kangaroo Mother Care should begin as soon as possible after birth, be applied as continuous skin-to-skin contact to the extent that this is possible and appropriate and continue for as long as appropriate."

Luong KC, Nguyen TL, Huynh Thi DH, *et al.* **Newly born low birthweight infants stabilise better in skin-to-skin contact than when separated from their mothers: a randomised controlled trial.** Acta Paediatr 2016;105:381-390

"Skin-to-skin contact was likely to be an optimal environment for neonates without life-threatening conditions who weighed 1500–2500 g at birth. By preventing instability that requires subsequent medical treatment, it may be life-saving in low-income countries."

BREASTFEEDING THE PREMATURE BABY: PART 2

Premature babies cannot start going to the breast until 34 weeks gestation?

This is simply not true. Experience and evidence (see references at bottom) from Scandinavia clearly show that babies can go to the breast well before 30 weeks gestation and as early as 27 weeks gestation. Not only can they go to the breast and latch on, but also, they can be getting milk from the breast by 28 to 30 weeks gestation, at least 4 or more weeks before in North America, they are even "allowed" to go to the breast.

In North America and elsewhere in the world, we believe, because it's true, that babies born at 24 weeks gestation and even earlier can be kept alive and leave hospital in reasonably good shape, but we just cannot believe a baby can go to the breast before 34 weeks gestation. How can that be?

High tech neonatology

Well, saving a baby of 24 weeks gestation is "high tech" and we really believe in "high tech" and admittedly, it was thought impossible only a few years ago that a 24 week gestation baby could survive.

"High tech" proves humans are above the other animals, and *neonatologists,* oh, they are superior beings, not quite gods, but just below, at the level of archangels, perhaps. But breastfeeding is "low tech", so "who cares?", "not interesting" and therefore *breastfeeding* is generally ignored (though *breastmilk,* which was a long time ignored as inferior, is now back in fashion, and ready for it? "High tech"). And what we believed about premature babies and breastfeeding 50 years ago, well, no point in looking any further, it's all the same, doesn't change. In fact, we believed that breastmilk was "low tech", (after all, made by women, so... must I say more?).

And then we started to find out more: that breastmilk made by the mother of a premature baby was tailor made for the needs of the premature, different than the milk of a mother of a baby born at term; we learned that breastmilk contains all sorts of very important compounds we never suspected even existed just a few years ago; for example, lysozyme (an enzyme, not so new actually, that attacks bacteria and kills them by destroying their cell wall), mucins, stem cells, lactadherin, bifidus factor, milk fat globule membranes, human milk oligosaccharides and *many* others. And probably many others are yet to be discovered.

And so, breastmilk became high tech and worthy of interest, *especially* by formula companies who realized the marketing potential immediately. But *breastfeeding*? Still "low tech" and is believed, wrongly, not worth thinking about. After all, breastmilk in a bottle is just as good as breastfeeding when the baby is actually getting milk directly from the breast. So why bother our heads about making sure the baby breastfeeds?

Except it's not true. Breastmilk in a bottle is not at all like breastmilk received from a warm, soft breast of a caring mother. Breastfeeding is a relationship, a close, physical and emotional relationship between two people usually in love. Bottle feeding is, well, bottle feeding.

Oh, yes, I forgot. Premature babies "need" "fortified" breastmilk, so we cannot have the mothers breastfeed. "High tech" wins over "low tech" again. But do babies all need "fortified" breastmilk?

But why 34 weeks?

But where does such an idea come from that a baby must be at least 34 weeks gestation before he can breastfeed? The answer depends on thinking breastfeeding and bottle feeding are essentially the same. It is said that bottle fed babies started on bottles before about 34 weeks gestation will have apneas (breathing stopped) and bradycardias (slow heart rate) as a result of bottle feeding. And we all know that bottle feeding is just like breastfeeding, breasts being just a softer bottle. NOT true. Bottle feeding is *not* just like breastfeeding, but we seem to believe it is. Thus, if babies younger than 34 weeks gestation have apneas and bradycardias while drinking from a bottle, they would likely have them while drinking from the breast. NOT true.

Breastfeeding is not bottle feeding and even if it's breastmilk in the bottle does not make bottle feeding like breastfeeding. Unlike what many neonatologists seem to believe, **breastfeeding does not take more energy** than bottle feeding and does not tire the baby out or cause the baby to fall asleep at the breast from fatigue or that babies fall asleep at the breast because they are "lazy". That is an error based on the observation that babies do tend to fall asleep at the breast even though when they come off the breast they show they are still hungry. But they don't fall asleep because they are tired or that breastfeeding takes up a lot of energy. They fall asleep because babies respond to the flow of milk from the breast. If the flow of milk is slow, the young baby tends to fall asleep at the breast.

The same is true of pacifiers, which are such a bad idea, but are frequently used in the neonatal intensive care units (NICUs). The baby is likely to fall asleep with the pacifier in his mouth because there is no flow. In some NICUs, the pacifier is actually taped in place, because when the baby falls asleep, the pacifier will usually fall out of the baby's mouth, and the baby will wake up and the idea that a premature baby must sleep is very much ingrained in NICU "thinking".

And why does the milk flow slow down when the baby is breastfeeding? Because, in most NICUs, we do not teach mothers **how to latch babies on**, and we don't teach them the simple useful "trick" of **breast compression**.

It is generally said in lactation consultant "circles" that babies do or do not transfer milk well. So, for example, "The baby is not gaining weight well because he is not transferring milk well." Well, in fact, babies don't transfer milk. **Mothers transfer milk**.

But the notion that it is the baby who "transfers milk" leads to the false conclusion that breastfeeding is hard work, that the baby has to use up a lot of energy in order to suck milk out of the breast. And this is even more so for a premature baby who has "undeveloped cheek muscles". Babies use their cheek muscles to pull milk out of the breast? None of the previous statements is true. **Babies respond to milk flow**. If milk flow is rapid and relatively consistent, the

241

baby usually stays awake and drinks the milk. If milk flow slows, the baby stops drinking and may only "nibble". And the flow of milk slows quickly because in most NICUs mothers are not taught **good latching on** and are not taught **breast compression**

The mother **in a video on** *www.ibconline.ca is using breast compression to increase the flow of milk to the baby who is only a few days old.*

Thus, premature babies in North America are not allowed to start breastfeeding until 34 weeks gestation, while at least some premature babies in Scandinavia can start at 27 weeks gestation. That makes no sense at all. And it is "obvious", also, that mothers should not keep the baby feeding at the breast "too long", thus tiring the baby out.

Another "obvious", but *incorrect* conclusion, is that babies need to be fed or supplemented by bottle, as everyone seems to believe that the bottle is less tiring. But that is believed only because we are used to the bottle. Supplementation can be done at the breast with a **lactation aid** which is the best way *if supplementation is necessary*, but also by open cup.

We have a video on www.ibconline.ca which shows a lactation aid at the breast to supplement a baby. Note that the baby falls asleep when the flow of milk slows but wakes up and sucks vigorously when the flow of milk, given by **lactation aid at the breast,** *increases. The baby was not tired and therefore fell asleep; the flow of milk was slow, and the baby fell asleep because the flow of milk was slow. When the flow increased, the baby woke up.*

Here are a few articles showing that babies can start going to the breast well before 34 weeks gestation. The comments below the reference are exact quotes from the article.

Blaymore JA, Ferguson AE, Morales Y, Liebling JA, Oh W, Vohr BR. **Breastfeeding Infants Who Were Extremely Low Birth Weight.** *Pediatrics*1997;100(6).

"Results. The infants demonstrated a higher oxygen saturation and a higher temperature during breastfeeding than during bottle feeding and were less likely to desaturate to <90% oxygen during breastfeeding. Mean weight gain was greater during bottle feeding than during breastfeeding (31 vs 9 g).

Conclusions. Breastfeeding the ELBW infant is desirable from a standpoint of improved physiologic responses, but such practice requires breastfeeding support and possible supplementation to optimize weight gain."

Hedberg Nyqvist K, Ewald U. **Infant and maternal factors in the development of breastfeeding behaviour and breastfeeding outcome in preterm infants.** *Acta Pædiatr* 1999;88:1194-203

"In conclusion, low gestational age at birth was associated with early emergence of efficient breastfeeding behaviour and a high incidence of full breastfeeding."

Nyqvist KH, Sjödén P-O, Ewald U. **The development of preterm infants' breastfeeding behavior.** *Early Human Development* 1999;55:247-264

"Irrespective of PMA (post menstrual age), the infants responded by rooting and sucking on the first contact with the breast. Efficient rooting, areolar grasp and latching on were observed at 28 weeks, and repeated bursts of >10 sucks and maximum bursts of >30 sucks at 32 weeks. Nutritive sucking appeared from 30.6 weeks. Sixty-seven infants were breastfed at discharge. Fifty-seven of them established full breastfeeding at a mean PMA of 36.0 weeks (33.4–40.0 weeks). Their early sucking behavior is interpreted as the result of learning, enhanced by contingent stimuli. We therefore suggest that guidelines for initiation of breastfeeding in preterm infants should be based on cardiorespiratory stability, irrespective of current maturity, age or weight."

Nyqvist KH, **Early attainment of breastfeeding competence in very preterm infants.** *Acta Pædiatrica* 2008;97:776-781

"Very preterm infants have the capacity for early development of oral motor competence that it sufficient for establishment of full breastfeeding at a low postmenstrual age."

BREASTFEEDING THE PREMATURE BABY: PART 3

What about "fortifiers"?

We will start off by saying that when I (Dr Jack Newman) finished my pediatric training at the Hospital for Sick Children in Toronto in 1981, I was a believer, more or less, in the way we did things with regard to breastfeeding the babies in the neonatal intensive care unit (NICU). It was obvious that we were putting obstacles in the way of mothers and babies, ensuring breastfeeding failure for most. The illnesses these babies had, such as respiratory distress syndrome of the premature (RDS), usually requiring ventilator support because of their immature lungs. Another common illness, necrotizing enterocolitis (NEC), which could lead to perforation of the baby's gut, also made breastfeeding difficult if not impossible for most mothers and their babies. While the babies were being mechanically ventilated, it was assumed that babies could not be breastfed or even be held in **skin to skin contact**. Necrotizing enterocolitis, if it occurs, does still require any oral feeding to be suspended, but we now know that **breastfeeding and even breastmilk decrease the risk of NEC**.

On top of that, the restrictions on the access mothers had to their babies were a large factor in the difficulties the mothers and babies ran into. Mothers were not allowed access to their babies during physician rounds, or if a baby in the same room was undergoing a procedure, and during nursing shift changes. Okay, no mothers in the room when the physicians were doing work rounds, fair enough, because of patient confidentiality. But many other reasons seemed good enough reasons to keep the mothers away from their babies.

And so, I thought, well, it's unfortunate, but there is nothing to be done. The thinking at the time was that saving the babies' life somehow prevented them being in skin to skin contact and breastfeeding as if the two were mutually exclusive. And, of course, we agree that saving the baby's life came first. As it turns out, very good work from Columbia (the country, not the university in New York City) and Scandinavia has shown that we can do everything to save the baby's life while, at the same time, encouraging mothers to do skin to skin contact and Kangaroo Mother Care and as a result help get the mother and baby breastfeeding successfully.

245

The thinking, in those days, came about as a result of considering breastfeeding as "extra", not vital, a bonus that the mother and baby can have, when and if the baby was well enough and big enough, but only then. However, in spite of the many studies demonstrating, without doubt, the benefits of Kangaroo Mother Care on the general wellbeing of the premature baby (and, incidentally, of full term), including the increased success of breastfeeding, many neonatal intensive care units have just not come on board. "What we've always done works well" seems to be the mindset, and "Please don't confuse me with facts".

These chapters **Breastfeeding the premature baby Parts 1,and 2** discuss some of the advances in the care and breastfeeding of premature babies that occurred over the last 35 or more years.

My experience in Africa

My first "real" job after finishing my training was as a pediatrician in the "Black Homeland" of the Transkei, an artificial country made to advance the Apartheid policy of the Republic of South Africa. Any Black Africans not supporting the economy of South Africa (by working at jobs frequently not substantially different from slavery) were forced to live in several scattered, generally very poor areas, where the land was infertile, rainfall sparse and no source of any sort of riches at all, not even mineral wealth for which South Africa is known.

I was the only pediatrician in the "country" where a study of the infant mortality rate (death before 1 year of age) was outlined by an epidemiologist not long after I arrived. He presented the results just tabulated that showed that 250 or so of every 1000 babies born in the Transkei died before the age of a year.

Part of my responsibilities as the pediatrician was to manage the "special care" unit. The unit was very poorly equipped compared to the ones of my experience in Toronto, and we not infrequently had 3 or 4 premature babies in the same incubator (they seemed to keep each other warmer, lying side by side, than the frequently malfunctioning incubators). There were no infant ventilators in the hospital at all. The mothers did stay with the babies much more than what I was used to in Toronto, but most had other children at home and so this made their being there most of the day difficult. When they could stay, they slept on the floor in an adjoining room and would come to breastfeed their babies whenever the babies showed readiness to feed.

And to my surprise, though formula and bottles were not allowed in the hospital, I had somehow expected that premature formula would be available for the premature babies, as "medicine", so to speak. But no, "No formula meant no formula".

In my training, I was taught the idea that premature babies should grow at the same rate as they would have, had they stayed in the uterus. So, what could I do? I "knew" that breastmilk alone could not make babies grow at the desired rate. How did I know this? I was taught this and believed it, just as many doctors believe the not always unspoken message in their training that breastfeeding cannot make even full term babies grow at the desired rate. Yes, such doctors are not rare.

It should be mentioned at the outset that one of the flaws of getting babies to gain at "intrauterine growth rate" is that overall gain in weight does not necessarily mean that the babies are actually getting the nutrients they need. Weight gain is a very crude measure of what adequate nutrition is. So, for example, lots of weight gain in a developing premature baby may mean that much of that weight is actually fat, not necessarily lung growth or brain growth. The notion that premature babies, once out of the uterus should grow as if they were still in the uterus is based on no science at all, but really based on "It seems like a good idea". But studies show that the push for more weight gain often leads to long term problems such as overweight, **higher blood pressure**, **higher cholesterol** and **insulin resistance** in adolescents born before term.

Furthermore, nobody knew in 1981 at Toronto's Hospital for Sick Children whether babies should be fed enterally (through the intestinal tract) for the first 7 to 10 days. The opinion shifted back and forth and sometimes every month,

247

depending on which neonatologist was in charge for that month. "Fasting" the babies for 7 to 10 days is part of the reason for the enthusiastic introduction of fortifiers, to catch up on what the baby didn't get during that time. It is now believed that **early enteral feeding** is a good thing.

How could I get the premature babies to gain weight at the intrauterine rate?

I couldn't use formula; I couldn't use a relatively new technique, new at the time, that is, called "total parenteral nutrition" which was a way of getting nutrients into the baby with an intravenous infusion of nutrients. It was beyond the money available, in a health system starved for funds for adequate care of anyone, never mind premature babies. And we didn't have the expertise to make up the solutions and monitor the results.

So, I decided that instead of using the standard amounts of milk given to babies in affluent countries, I would give the premature babies *more breastmilk*.

Usually it is said that premature babies can take only up to 180 to 200 cc/kg/day fluid total in 24 hours (by enteral methods + intravenous). In some neonatal intensive care units (NICUs), the "rule" is even less fluid. If the baby is receiving intravenous fluids, that may mean little is given into the intestinal tract. In an NICU this *may* make sense since the babies are sick, often on ventilators and some babies on ventilators may go into heart failure if they receive larger amounts of fluid. If the baby goes into heart failure while on a ventilator it may become difficult to wean the baby from the ventilator. But, the well premature baby *can* take more, especially if given by **continuous gastric tube feeding**, drop by drop into the baby's stomach.

We started gingerly, slowly increasing the amount of milk the baby received. We ended up giving 300+ cc/kg/day (4.6+ ounces/pound/day) with no trouble except occasionally babies would get watery bowel movements. But what is the meaning of watery bowel movements in the exclusively breastfed (or breastmilk fed) baby? This could be normal with large volumes of breastmilk and is seen in full term, healthy babies as well.

In any case, the babies thrived, we had no evidence of osteopenia (low levels of calcium in the bones). Okay, admittedly, these were babies who were not very sick, not like many babies we frequently see in NICUs in North America and Europe. They were generally bigger (babies born at 24 weeks gestation rarely, if ever, survived). But the point is that we could make them grow at rates that were similar to how they would have grown had they stayed in the uterus. And we did it with breastmilk only.

With the limited numbers of laboratory tests we could use, the babies were fine and biochemically did not show signs of osteopenia except unusually, but then we could add calcium and phosphorus, not a fortifier, to the milk.

What is the lesson for NICUs in resource-rich countries?

I think we can say a few things:

1. Problems with breastfeeding babies in the NICU are very much caused by current NICU routines and practices and by the fact that breastfeeding is presumed, in many hospitals, not to be a priority, too much work and often even seen as impossible. Vital steps are not taken to ensure premature babies have opportunities to breastfeed.

Here is an email from a mother: "One day my baby was skin to skin with me and she latched on my breast and began breastfeeding. A nurse noticed and said I should not allow her to do that as she is not yet strong enough. Since then, every day when I went to have my one hour of skin to skin contact with my baby, I would let her breastfeed in secret and made sure the nurse did not see us." The notion that **breastfeeding is tiring or too much work is wrong**. But even more so, who decides about breastfeeding: NICU staff or the mothers?

Here is a list of NICU routines that make breastfeeding premature babies difficult and promote the "need" for fortifiers:

- No **skin to skin contact** of the mother and baby or skin to skin contact being limited to an hour or so a day. But Kangaroo Mother Care is much of the day, not a couple of hours.

- The notion that babies need to first learn to bottle feed before they can be allowed to breastfeed.

- The routine use of pacifiers presumed to "teach babies how to suck".

- The routine use of **nipple shields** thought to be necessary and helpful for premature babies and the bizarre notion that a baby gets more milk through a nipple shield than latched on directly to the breast. If the baby actually does get more milk through a nipple shield than directly from the breast, it means the baby's latch to the breast is not good. Studies that have "shown" that babies get more milk through a nipple shield usually do not take into consideration whether the latch is good or not, because the staff and mothers usually have not been taught how to know. It is simply assumed that if the baby has the breast in his mouth and makes sucking movements, the baby must be getting milk. And it's just not true.

All these routines, combined with the notion that faster weight gain is better, pushes the use of fortifiers in the NICUs. Marketing by the formula companies, as well as formula sponsored conferences with "breastfeeding experts" reinforce the general belief that the fortifiers are necessary. And parents also agree as weight gain is linked to their being able to take the baby home.

Are "human milk fortifiers" made of human milk?

There is an issue that arises when the "fortifiers" are called "human milk fortifiers". This gives the impression to many parents that the babies are not getting formula, but that is exactly what fortifiers are: formula. Mothers of premature babies who come to our clinic for help with breastfeeding often say that their babies received only breastmilk when they were in the NICU, presumably because the "fortifiers" are called "human milk fortifiers".

2. "Fortifiers" just like any other formula are frequently overused, used unnecessarily and for much too long, without proof that they are necessary. "Fortifiers" are not always necessary for premature babies. They are presumed necessary because formulas are the accepted, "scientific" way to feed babies and breastmilk and breastfeeding are seen as unreliable. This assumption also causes health professionals not to prioritize breastfeeding and not to look for ways in which babies can be breastfed exclusively or receive only breastmilk.

3. In some NICUs, babies of 34 weeks gestation and even older, weighing 1500 grams (3lb 5oz) or even more at birth are routinely given "fortified" breastmilk. This is usually completely unnecessary especially if the mother has the baby in Kangaroo Mother Care (skin to skin much of the day), is taught **how to put the baby to the breast** so that the baby has a good latch and gets more milk while at the same time preventing the mother from getting sore. Mothers should also be taught **breast compression** to get the baby to take in more milk.

It is the pre- and post- weights that are done without teaching the mother the above important techniques, while at the same time believing that pre- and post-weights actually tell us something, that often results in the "need" for "fortification". Another reason is the idea, strongly touted in the NICUs, that babies must be fed every three hours and calculating down to the last millilitre the amount they must get at each feeding.

4. In some NICUs, mothers are being told that they must "fortify" their breastmilk until the baby is 10 months old. This is madness. This is an approach that truly speaks volumes about how little confidence some neonatologists and other pediatricians have in breastmilk and breastfeeding.

5. "Fortification" of breastmilk means that a significant amount of the breastmilk that is given the baby does not come directly from the breast. And usually that means by nasogastric feedings and/or bottles. The result is that most mothers in resource-rich countries go home with their babies not breastfeeding, though the babies may be getting some breastmilk.

Here are some of the reasons why breastfeeding in the NICU is difficult: Babies are fed according to a schedule and they are fed prescribed amounts of milk.

Mothers are allowed to come in and feed the baby who may have been overfed just before the mother arriving (a schedule is a schedule). And so, the baby is fast asleep and difficult to wake up just when the mother is there to feed the baby. The mother is then told she is disturbing the baby who needs to sleep to grow and she should put the baby back into the incubator.

6. Very tiny premature babies may need extra calories or calcium and phosphorus in the first days or weeks, but this does not mean they need fortifiers made from cow's milk and it does not mean they should not be breastfed as soon as the baby can start oral feedings. Fortifiers made from human milk have been available for many years. True, they are more expensive, even though the one company I am aware of does not pay the breastmilk donors for their milk. But if "fortification" were not practically routine, the overall cost of "fortifiers" to the hospital would decrease if used only when necessary.

7. In fact, "fortifiers" made from breastmilk, either donated or the mother's own milk, could be made in any hospital. For extra calories, the fat in the milk could be skimmed off and added to the mother's own milk and given to the baby. Depending on the baby's blood levels of alkaline phosphatase (which suggests that the baby's bones may or may not be "thinning out") calcium and phosphorus could easily be added to the mother's milk. It would be important not to use bottles when the baby is receiving fortifiers as there is a superior method to do so if supplementation is truly necessary: using the **lactation aid at the breast**.

We have a video on www.ibconline.ca which shows how to supplement a baby at the breast with a lactation aid.

BREASTFEEDING A TODDLER

There is no lack of "opinions" about the breastfeeding of a toddler. Almost everyone has something to say. "If he's old enough to ask for it, he's too old." "If he's got teeth, it's nature's way of saying, it's time to stop." And not rarely: "Breastfeed a 1 year old? That's disgusting." And even health professionals get into the act. Here, "words of wisdom" from a French child psychiatrist, as quoted in Le Soir, a French language Belgian newspaper, on November 29, 2003: "One does not share the breast: to extend breastfeeding past 7 months is without doubt sexual abuse". "...without doubt sexual abuse".

How do people who say such things develop such strange notions? Breastfeeding into toddlerhood has been the norm in much of the world until very recently.

Here are some quotes on breastfeeding a child older than a baby, from various works of literature

"On Lammas-eve at night shall she be fourteen;
That shall she, marry: I remember it well.
'Tis since the earthquake now eleven years;
And she was wean'd, I never shall forget it,
Of all the days of the year, upon that day;"

William Shakespeare. Romeo and Juliet. (Juliet weaned at 3 years old).

"And have you any children?"
"I've had four; I've two living—a boy and a girl. I weaned her last carnival."
"How old is she?"
"Why, two years old."
"Why did you nurse her so long?"
"It's our custom; for three fasts..."

Leo Tolstoy. Anna Karenina

"Only seldom was a whimper heard from one of the four children, all of whom, from the six-month-old infant to the six-year-old Amanda, were fed from Louise's breast.

"Never again, never in the future that dawned later on, were we so sated. We were suckled and suckled. Always superabundance was flowing into us. Never any question of enough is enough or let's not overdo it. Never were we given a pacifier and told to be reasonable. It was always suckling time.

"There must be reasons why we men are so hipped on breasts as if we'd all been weaned too soon."

Günter Grass. The Flounder

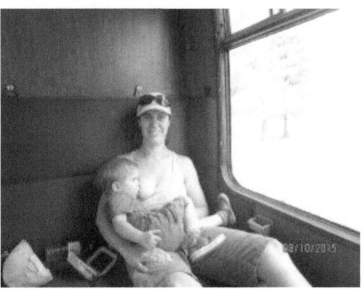

A toddler breastfeeding in a train. A perfectly normal thing to do.

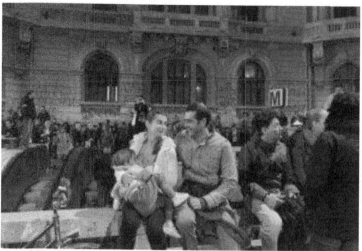
*A toddler being breastfed in a public space with many people
around without getting their knickers in a knot.*

Why does it even matter to those who say such things as "If he's old
enough to ask for it..."?

What business is it of theirs? Despite what people might say, accusing us of
shaming mothers who don't breastfeed (we don't), haranguing mothers at the
shopping mall about bottle feeding their babies (we don't), telling our patients
at the International Breastfeeding Centre that formula is poison (we don't), why
can't people just shut up about a mother who breastfeeds a toddler? Except
maybe to tell her it's a beautiful thing she is doing.

Here are our thoughts on why it matters to so many people

First of all, because in our society breasts are perceived as sexual playthings
only. And, of course, the breast does have an erotic purpose. But so does the
mouth; so, should we cover our mouths in public because the mouth has an
erotic purpose as well? We accept that the mouth is for eating and the mouth
also has a sexual or erotic side. But we can't seem to accept that the breast is
not *only* sexual.

255

As a result, we accept, grudgingly, that a baby breastfeeds, but a toddler? That's a little *too* disturbing. That's like having sex with children. And that's where the comments in the first paragraph of this chapter come from, the disgust at the notion of having sex with children. Except that breastfeeding a toddler, get ready for it, is *not* having sex with that toddler.

Sigmund Freud helped propagate the idea that breastfeeding a toddler is somehow not right. Freud believed that children go through several developmental stages, starting from 0 to 1 year with the oral stage, followed by the anal stage which lasts few years, to be followed by a latent stage... He believed, *without any real proof,* that you cannot be in two different stages at the same time, and it is a sign of "delayed development" if a child is still showing signs of being in the oral stage after a year. In other words, still breastfeeding. Psychiatrists are aware of this because they study Freud, but the rest of us have basically forgotten about this declaration of Freud's while at the same time believing it.

Well, it's okay to breastfeed after a year. It's fine and perfectly normal to breastfeed until the child can ask for it and even discuss how much he or she loves it. It's *not* disgusting. The only disgusting part of this whole issue is the reactions of too many people who find breastfeeding a toddler disgusting.

Many doctors (and nutritionists) believe there is nothing in breastmilk after a year (some say 6 months)

If there is nothing in breastmilk after a year, then what's the point of breastfeeding? Here is where the mother is blamed. "She's doing it only for herself", for keeping her toddler a baby and not developing normally, and incredibly, for some sort of sexual pleasure.

The thing is, that breastfeeding is so much more than breastmilk. It is a relationship, a **close, intimate physical and emotional relationship** between two people who are generally in love with each other.

In spite of there being a ton of proof that breastmilk still contains, protein, fat, carbohydrate, immune factors, and growth factors and much more after a year and after 3 years and even longer, many doctors and nutritionists persist in this idea that breastmilk contains nothing after a certain time after birth.

In fact, after a year, breastmilk still contains the long chained polyunsaturated fatty acids (DHA and ARA) that the formula companies like to imply they invented. The antibodies and multiple other immune factors that help resist infection are still there, some in greater quantities than during the first few months after birth. The various growth factors (factors which stimulate the development of various organ systems) are still present in the breastmilk. Growth factors present in breastmilk aid in the maturation of the brain, the gut, and the immune system, as well as other systems. **Breastmilk always contains stem cells, alpha lactalbumin which, when exposed to stomach acid, changes into HAMLET (human alpha lactalbumin made lethal to tumour cells), and so much more.**

How do doctors conclude that there is nothing in breastmilk after a year?

We can only guess, but we think the guess has a solid basis in fact.

It is not rare for a small number of older babies and toddlers to spend long periods on the breast and yet not gain weight. This occurs, usually, because the mother has had **a significant decrease in her milk supply**. The baby is sucking on the breast and without getting very much milk at all. Most health professionals do not seem to know how to look at a baby or toddler at the breast and know if the baby is drinking milk or not. They believe that if the baby is latched on and making sucking movements, he must be getting milk which is not necessarily true. So, they assume there is nothing in breastmilk after a year or any arbitrary period time after birth. But this is patently false to anyone who knows something about breastfeeding.

We have a video on www.ibconline.ca which shows the baby is receiving lots of milk. You can tell because of the pause in the chin as he opens his mouth to the maximum. Each suck is open-pause-close. That pause says "I just got a mouth full of milk". The longer the pause, the more milk the baby received.

Not gaining much from the breast yet refuses to eat food?

In some cases, the baby spends long periods of time at the breast, is not getting much milk, is not gaining weight, perhaps even losing weight, and yet, refuses to eat food. How can that be? How can a baby who is obviously not getting enough milk to gain weight or is even losing weight, why would that baby refuse food which is offered to him? Hungry people, babies included, gobble up food.

We believe that the mother's milk supply has decreased to the point where these babies are, in fact, on a low-calorie diet. It's not that there is nothing in breastmilk; it's that the baby is not getting breastmilk, at least not very much of it. So, they develop ketosis, a situation that several fad diets try to induce in the dieter. Don't eat much, you develop ketones in your blood and you don't feel hungry.

But why do the babies stay on the breast for long periods if they are ketotic? *Because breastfeeding is more than nutrients and calories.* **Breastfeeding gives the baby security, comfort and, yes, love.** So, they stay on the breast and suck and suck and don't get much in the way of nutrients, but they do get comfort.

Most pediatricians will tell the mother she must stop breastfeeding and the baby will start to eat. In fact, that's not necessarily true. Yes, some will start eating, but not all, so it's dangerous to just stop breastfeeding, because some babies may become dangerously dehydrated and malnourished. They may then be hospitalized for nasogastric feedings and then they will start to eat food as well once they get a lot of calories. More proof that there is nothing in breastmilk? The fact that health professionals generally have no practical knowledge of breastfeeding makes such wrong conclusions possible.

But hospital is not necessarily a safe place for a malnourished baby or toddler. And this approach ends the breastfeeding and that is a significant price to pay. And it's not necessary to hospitalize the child or stop breastfeeding.

What can be done? **Increase the baby's intake of breastmilk at the breast**! When the baby gets more milk from the breast, the ketosis decreases and disappears, and the baby starts to feel hungry and starts to eat food and at the same time continues breastfeeding. This is a better solution. We frequently use **domperidone** in this situation and it works. The mother's milk increases, the baby gets more milk, the ketosis goes away, and the baby starts eating food as well as breastfeeds.

It should be pointed out that even if everything is going well with the breastfeeding, doctors will frequently tell mothers to stop breastfeeding because "there are no further benefits for the baby". This of course says volumes about that doctor's understanding of breastfeeding in general but also breastfeeding the toddler.

Please see: Health Canada's statement on feeding the baby 6 to 24 months.
American Academy of Pediatrics statement on breastfeeding.
WHO recommendations on duration of breastfeeding.

And a few quotes from the World Health Organization:

"Breast-milk is also an important source of energy and nutrients in children aged 6–23 months."

"Breast-milk is also a critical source of energy and nutrients during illness."

"Longer durations of breastfeeding also contribute to the health and well-being of mothers: it reduces the risk of ovarian and breast cancer and helps space pregnancies."

STARTING BABIES ON FOOD

Modern medicine, in a worthwhile desire to avoid problems associated with poor eating habits, has developed rules about the feeding of food to babies that have made eating food a complicated, frightening and a tiresome exercise. These rules are even more complicated when parents must choose the "right foods" for their children, especially those still too young to choose for themselves.

Most paediatric societies, including the **Canadian Paediatric Society** and the **American Academy of Pediatrics**, agree with the **World Health Organization** statement that babies be breastfed exclusively for the first 6 months and that solids be started when the babies are 6 months old. This seems simple enough, not at all complicated. But on closer inspection and when we are trying to deal with the real world, some issues come up.

It should be emphasized that the **normal length of breastfeeding usually is about 3 – 5 years** and longer because toddlers and young children need breastfeeding not only for nutrition but also as a **relationship**.

It is worthwhile remembering that these statements by the WHO, the Canadian Paediatric Society and the American Academy of Pediatrics, as well as other pediatric societies around the world, are public health statements, and are true for most babies, but not necessarily for *all* babies. Perhaps we can say that the statements are an "ideal" approach to starting babies on food, but that there are times or babies for whom the statement may not be appropriate.

Unfortunately, too often, mothers writing us with regard to their baby seeming hungry, their baby who will turn 6 months of age in one week, will state, in response to our suggestion (**amongst others**) that the baby be started on food: "We plan to start him on food next week".

Is that what the WHO and other statements really suggest, that the baby be exactly 6 months, 182.5 days old, before starting food? We don't think so. What happens when it is a leap year?

Please see at the end of this chapter some unusual situations with regard to food, under the title of **Late onset decreased milk supply** and Ketosis.

Why would there be exceptions?

The obvious answer is that not all babies are the same; they reach developmental milestones at various times and parents watching for signs of the baby's readiness to eat food is more important than looking strictly at the calendar. The beginning of the baby's interest in food may vary, as does the timing of a baby's sitting up without support, saying words and independent walking.

It seems obvious that the baby should decide when he is ready to eat food and parents usually are quite aware that their baby starts to become interested in eating food.

By about four months of age, many babies are becoming interested in what their parents are eating. The baby, sitting in a high chair (at four months usually supported by pillows) or on one of his parent's lap while the parent is eating, may follow with fascinated interest the progress of the spoon or fork from the plate to the parent's mouth. At about the same time, the baby is starting to develop the hand-eye coordination which will allow him to pick up food and other objects and put them into his mouth.

By about 6 months, many babies are trying to reach for food and many, if food is within reach, will try to take the food and put it into their mouth. This seems an appropriate time to start offering food to the baby.

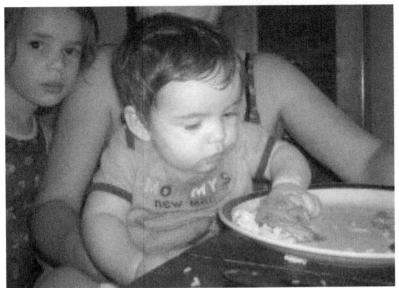

This baby is almost 6 months old, but not quite. He obviously is interested in eating. Should the parents wait until exactly 6 months?

However, some babies seem very anxious to start solids earlier than 6 months of age. Why should parents feel they must wait until the magical 6 months? So, starting earlier than 6 months, say, 5 months and 1 week, would be, in our opinion, perfectly appropriate, BUT, please see the paragraph on **late onset decreased milk supply**, below.

Starting at this age, however, depends on the baby's desire to start food, not the parents' desire to start "real food" as opposed to breastmilk (often put down as not "real food"). Grandparents, hoping that, finally, they can take part in the feeding the baby themselves, often imply that breastmilk is not "real food". Or, too often, unfortunately, due to a lack of confidence in breastfeeding, even if the baby is happy and gaining weight well.

A comment, though, about the 5 month and 1 week old baby being very interested in solids. Besides the importance of making sure he is still breastfeeding well and that the mother has not had a **decrease in her milk supply**, it is true that the baby may be happier with eating food. But it is more important that the possible problem of the decrease in milk supply be addressed. Breastfeeding is still the most important food at this time.

And, in a world where formula companies keep clamouring for food (their food product) and formula (their formula) to be introduced to babies earlier and earlier and where public policy of 6 months of exclusive breastfeeding is being questioned more and more, what should be reinforced in people's minds is that they keep breastfeeding exclusively for 6 months.

On the other hand, some babies may not show interest in food until, say, 7 months of age. Is it okay to wait? Sure. If all is going well with the baby's breastfeeding, then it's fine, no problem. Exclusive breastfeeding to 6 months is a guideline, a suggestion, a "best practice" perhaps, but not a law. If the baby is not quite ready to eat until 7 months, say, what's wrong with that?

The baby shows signs of being ready; let's start the baby eating food

Your baby is around six months old and seems ready to eat food. What foods should you start offering him? It's not really complicated: basically: the same food that the parents eat with a very few exceptions (see below). There is no need at all for special foods for healthy, thriving babies of 6 months of age.

By six months of age, babies are interested in eating the same food as the rest of the family. Why? Well, they have become social beings and they want to participate in the same activities as their parents and siblings. This is usually pretty obvious to parents. Babies are different at 6 months than they were at 2 months, say. Also, they mimic the adults' behaviour more. That's how babies learn, by mimicking adult and older sibling behaviour.

The babies in the photos below are eating what the parents are eating, in the top photo, chewing a chicken bone and why not? In the photo below the first, the baby is eating a bit of meat.

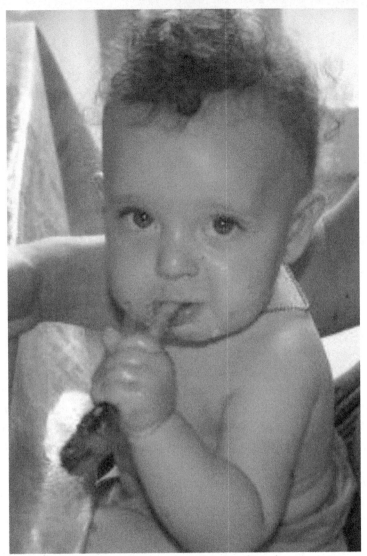

This baby, about 8 months old, is chewing on a chicken bone. Better than a teething ring, no?

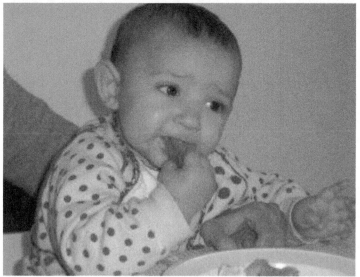

This baby is also about 8 months old. He is eating meat. And why not? Same food as his parents.

And this photo below? Baby and mother eating the same food.

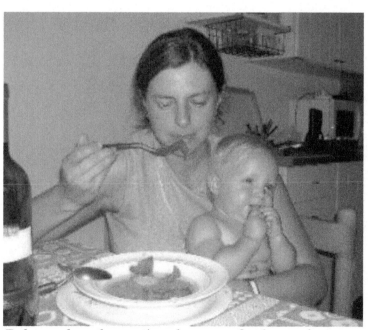

Baby and mother eating the same food, together. The baby is eating without help, not being spoon fed.

Eating has always been a social and family event, at least until recently. "Give us this day our daily bread" with the family around the table is no longer the norm, it seems. But maybe, if we reinforce the social nature of eating by not feeding, babies and children differently from the rest of the family, perhaps the family all eating together will return as a normal way of eating.

As you start offering food to your baby, you can also give him water to drink from an open cup; no need for special cups or sippy cups which are essentially modified bottles.

And you know what? The baby can and should be eating without help. Of course, somebody needs to be with him when he's eating, but the baby does not need to be spoon fed. He can pick up the food and eat it without help, with his hands. If you don't like messes, it's time to get over that. Babies are anything but neat, as you already know.

The photos below show babies who don't really care if they make a mess. Perhaps the parents should not care either. If you do care, put plastic around the high chair.

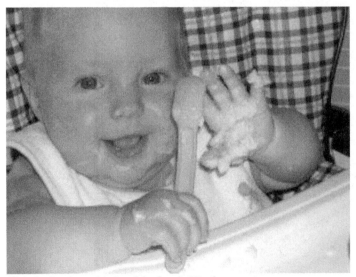

This baby is enjoying his food. He does not care much about neatness and cleanliness. Neither

should you. Let him enjoy his food.

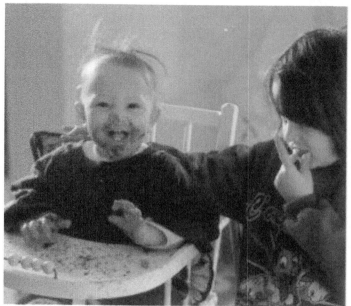

This baby covered the table of the high chair and much of himself with the food. But he is very happy, no?

What about breastfeeding at this point?

Once a baby is six months old, all attention shifts to "food" and very little attention is paid to breastfeeding. And not infrequently people believe, wrongly, that breastmilk no longer contains the necessary nutrients the baby needs.

There is a widespread notion amongst physicians and nutritionists that there is "nothing in breastmilk" after about 6 months. This is patently false. See below in the section **Late onset decreased milk supply** and Ketosis for more information.

Breastfeeding can and should continue after the first six months and *food is added to breastfeeding*. Food does not substitute for breastfeeding at this point and breastfeeding is not a supplement to food; breastfeeding is the main food. If problems with breastfeeding appear at this point, when your baby is 9 or 12 months or older, the problems can be overcome, and it is not a sign that your baby is "**self-weaning**". A baby does not "self-wean" before the age of 2.5 or 3 years of age. The time between 6 months and 2 years serves to give the baby time to learn to eat the food adults eat and to establish breastfeeding and food as two important sides of normal eating.

Introducing gluten

A big deal has been made about babies needing to be exposed to gluten early in life, in order to prevent the development of coeliac disease. According to two fairly sketchy studies, babies have a decreased incidence of coeliac disease later in life if they are exposed to gluten containing foods between 4 and 7 months of age (not before 4 months and not after 7 months).

But these studies did not prove anything. And in fact, they didn't find the children had a decreased incidence of coeliac disease. One US study found that babies started on food AFTER 4 months of age were better off than babies started on food BEFORE 4 months of age. One Swedish study did not include the question of whether babies were breastfed or not. And there have been many studies since then showing that there was no relationship between the timing of gluten introduction and coeliac disease.

In any case, there is no need for commercial infant cereals to expose the baby to gluten (see the photo below).

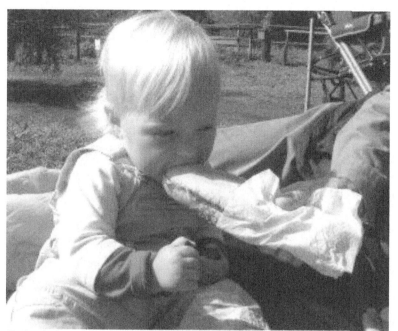

Baby being exposed to gluten in a tastier manner than with infant cereals. No need for cereals, which are truly overrated foods.

Foods your baby really doesn't need

Formula, "follow-on" formula (also called "follow-up" formula and "toddler" formula)

Your six month old breastfed baby who is learning to eat food does not need to start drinking any kind of formula or "special" formula. And definitely a six month old baby eating food does not need "follow-on" formula or "toddler formula", no matter how convincing the advertising, even if he was receiving formula before he started on food. When the baby starts eating food, he can now do without formula supplements if he eats enough food. There is no point at which your healthy breastfed baby who is also eating a variety of foods, would need formula after the age of six months even if he was supplemented with formula during the first 6 months.

This is also not a time to introduce bottles. Breastfed babies should be learning to eat normal food and to drink from the open cups they will also be using later on in life.

Where does the notion that babies need these products come from? Well, as mentioned above, from advertising. Formula companies know where the money is. As Willie Sutton, an American bank robber, said when he was captured and asked why he robbed banks "That's where the money is". Of course, formula companies do not rob banks; they have easier prey: parents worried by all sorts of tactics suggesting their babies are not getting "good nutrition".

But also, there is the widespread idea in the minds of doctors that babies between 6 months and 2 years need 900 ml (30 oz) of milk in 24 hours. This is pure fantasy. Formulas are, essentially, liquefied solid foods. There is no advantage of follow-on formulas over normal food. If the parents want to give dairy products to the baby, then cheese or yogurt are just fine, and liquid milk is not necessary or desirable and even *undesirable* if given by bottle.

There remains the historical knowledge in older physicians' minds that too much cow's milk would result in bleeding from the intestines and anemia in the older baby. The picture of the fat, pale baby remains deep in their memories. So, no cow's milk; only formula. And breastfeeding? What happened to breastfeeding in this picture? Breastmilk does *not* cause bleeding from the intestines. Except, *rarely*, when there has been **late onset decreased milk supply**, and it's *not* breastmilk that causes the bleeding, but a *decrease* in the baby's intake of breastmilk that causes the bleeding. And the problem is corrected by increasing the intake of breastmilk by the baby.

A frequently made argument is that if the family cannot afford "good, nutritious food", the baby would do well with the follow on formula. But in fact, the cost of follow on formula is greater than most good nutritious food. Moreover, the baby can and should continue to be breastfed, thus ensuring "good nutrition".

Commercial infant cereals

If the baby is eating commercial infant cereals, it is clear to him that he is not eating what the rest of the family is eating, so why give him this food?

Infant cereals are touted as good first foods for babies, but they really aren't. They are not even okay, in our opinion, partly because the rest of the family is not eating that stuff and partly because they are basically introducing "instant fast food" to the baby. Furthermore, the commercial cereals do not taste very good at all.

Commercial infant cereals were introduced into the mass market in North America in the 1920s and 1930s. Parents were encouraged to give these foods from very early on, from the baby's age of 2 or 3 months and sometimes even earlier. Besides making money for the manufacturer, they were promoted as providing the baby with "easily digestible" food, containing important elements the manufacturers claimed were not easily available in other foods babies were first given. And this worry about the baby missing out on "not easily available nutrients" has been with the parents ever since.

Back in the 1920s and 1930s, with more and more pediatricians pushing formula feeding as "scientific infant feeding", often to the exclusion of breastfeeding, infant cereals were "nutritional insurance" against nutrients missing in formulas at the time. Especially home-made formulas (1part cow's milk, 2 parts water, 1 tablespoon of corn syrup and less water and more corn syrup as the baby gets bigger).

These cereals, even the modern versions, tend to taste bland, at best, and bad, at worst. And they are expensive for what you get from a nutritional point of view. Indeed, the nutritional value of most commercial cereals is rather lacking. The only nutrient thought to be of possible potential value, but in truth serves only to market the product, is the iron that has been added. But, most of the iron, which is poorly absorbed, ends up in the baby's diaper. And because of the high levels of iron in the cereals, commercial cereals tend to be constipating.

Another brilliant marketing stratagem?

Let's add formula to infant cereal! Brilliant indeed, trying to convince parents that the cereals are "better than ever" and selling more formula at the same time. Win-win for the formula companies.

In fact, the "need" for iron has been overly exaggerated, based on the knowledge that breastmilk does not contain a lot of iron. Did nature mess up? What could possibly be the reason for "insufficient" amounts of iron in breastmilk?

It was assumed, on the basis of "nutritional theory", that because the concentration of iron in breastmilk is low, this was a bad thing. Exclusively breastfed, thriving babies are, it needs to be remembered and too often forgotten, the *physiological norm*.

They are meant to get iron from three sources – during the pregnancy, from blood transferred to the baby by the umbilical cord at birth and breastmilk which contains iron in a very absorbable form. And it is quite possible that the decrease in iron stores that occurs in the exclusively breastfed baby around 6 months of age actually has a beneficial effect in **preventing infection** in the baby when he starts food.

High levels of iron in the intestinal tract of a baby encourage the growth of pathogenic (disease causing) bacteria that need iron in order to multiply, thus increasing the risk of serious infection. Once the baby is six months old, he will start to eat food, but at an age where his immunity has developed to the point that he could fight off these infections, especially if he is still breastfeeding.

In any case, iron can be naturally found in **foods** other than infant cereals (to which it is added artificially), and often the absorption of the iron is more complete than from infant cereals.

The latest in selling parents useless foods for their babies

The infant food industry loses no opportunity to make money on the backs of parents who really want to do the best for their children. There is now available, a whole array of "special baby food" in "food pouches", and parents are being convinced that babies are to be started on "special food" first – blended vegetables, fruit and even whole meals. This includes special "teas" for babies, special baby cookies (with "vitamins") and even special pasta, ham and yogurt. So instead of being taught to eat normal food, babies are frequently transferred from one bottle to another sort of bottle (the pouch) and from one formula to another version of "formula". Popular in Europe is special "baby water". Coming to your local grocery store soon! And how much do they cost? 1.5 litres in Europe cost 1.75 euros ($2.60 Canadian, $2.09 US). For water!

With these food pouches babies can suck and feed themselves any time they want to eat, even when being pushed along in a stroller. Even at the dinner table, these pouches result in "different food for the baby", partly overcome, perhaps, by having the rest of the children eating from these pouches.

But these pouches have babies and young children sucking on a bottle, essentially. Lactation consultants have noted that babies who suck on these pouches more than occasionally actually breastfeed less well. And lactation consultants have seen several mothers develop **late onset sore nipples** which got better once they stopped the pouches.

And although individual pouches seem inexpensive, in fact they are not. A child eating food that comes from the family's plates, would eat for much less money than the cost of one of these pouches. And think about all these unrecyclable containers. Who is paying for them? Not the company, that's on the parents' bill.

Many of these pouches contain elevated quantities of sugar, which, finally, we are beginning to understand can contribute to childhood and adult overweight and obesity and diabetes type 2.

Health Canada states that babies older than 6 months should be drinking from an open cup, not a bottle and not sucking on a sippy cup. What is the difference between a food pouch and a sippy cup, or a bottle for that matter?

273

What foods should be avoided for a young baby?

The one group of foods that should be avoided are those that are called "choking hazards". The most notorious type of food going down "the wrong way" (into the lungs) was popcorn, though one wonders who would feed an 8 month old popcorn.

Health Canada recommends cutting up any food that is slippery and could potentially block the trachea (whole grapes, for example). Okay, makes sense. But Health Canada also recommends cutting blueberries in half. Really? Who is going to do that? "I just cut 5 blueberries in half and I think part of my finger is mixed in".

Late onset decreased milk supply, a significant problem for some mothers whose milk supply started off abundant and later decreased

In some cases of late onset decreased milk supply, the parents have reported that the baby was very interested in eating food well before the baby turned 6 months of age. This observation, in itself, may or may not be of significance because we tend to see late onset decreased milk supply around the same time that babies become interested, normally, in eating food. However, if we combine early interest in food plus the fact that the baby spends a lot of time sucking his fingers, or pulling at the breast, as well as other **symptoms mentioned in the chapter**, we think that, yes, in some cases the parents' observation does indeed go along with late onset decreased milk supply.

Ketosis

In other cases, when the mother's milk supply has decreased significantly, the baby may stay on the breast much of the day or have a pacifier in his mouth much of the day. The baby on the breast much of the day without gaining weight is often interpreted by those who do not know how to know the baby is drinking or not drinking at the breast, as: "there is no nutritional value to breastmilk after a certain age" often stated as after 6 months of age or after 1 year of age.

The real problem is that the baby is *not getting* much milk from the breast. What so many health professionals do not understand is that a baby is not drinking milk simply because the baby is latched on to the breast and making sucking motions with his mouth.

And yet, logically, it seems to make no sense that a baby not receiving enough milk to gain weight would refuse to eat solids. This is taken as proof positive by many pediatricians and nutritionists that there "is nothing in breastmilk after the first few months". But they can only say this because they do not watch the baby on the breast, and even if they did, they would not know what to watch for.

On the other hand, the mother is often told that the baby is using too much energy sucking all day long and using up the calories he gets from the breast. But this too is a misconception, based on the notion that babies "**transfer milk**". Babies don't transfer milk; mothers transfer milk. Babies, of course, do their part in the breastfeeding process, their sucking stimulates the milk to flow from the breast. The baby is not a passive vessel, after all.

But why would the baby refuse solids if he's gaining little or no weight? It is true that the baby is not getting a lot of nutrients and calories, not because there is nothing in breastmilk after the first few months but rather because the baby is not getting much milk, period. And this makes the baby *ketotic*, just as dieters on some fad diets, the purpose of which is to induce ketosis in the dieter. When you are ketotic, you lose your appetite. Thus, the baby has no interest in eating solids but continues on the breast because he gets **comfort and security from the breast**, another concept many health professionals still do not understand.

The other illogical deduction often made in such situations is that the baby is on the breast all the time, and thus filling up so much with the breastmilk that he's not hungry. But if the baby were really "filling up on breastmilk", the baby would be gaining weigh just fine because there are a lot of calories and nutrients in breastmilk, enough to make a baby double his birth weight in 3 to 4 months breastfeeding only. A baby is not getting milk from the breast just because he is latched on and making sucking motions.

INDUCING LACTATION

A person might wish to induce lactation if:

- They are adopting a baby

- They have a gestational carrier for their biological baby

- If they are in a relationship with woman who is pregnant and wishes to help in breastfeeding the baby

- Another relationship, often transgender, where one or both of the partners wishes to breastfeed

How can someone breastfeed if they have never been pregnant?

Our approach basically tries to make the body of the person inducing lactation "believe" that they are pregnant.

The hormonal milieu of the body during pregnancy compared to the non-pregnant state includes:

- High levels of estrogen

- High levels of progesterone

- High levels of prolactin

- High levels of human gonadotropin hormone

- High levels of other hormones

These hormones begin to rise with the onset of pregnancy. Each hormone has a role to play in the preparation of the breasts to make milk, with milk production starting about 16 weeks of pregnancy.

If a person has previously breastfed, this fact does increase the possibility of that person producing a full milk supply, but not necessarily so. Some persons inducing lactation have produced all the milk the baby needed, but we believe the majority do not.

What if I can't produce all the milk the baby needs?

It would be nice if you did, but please try to remember that breastfeeding is not just about milk and **breastfeeding is much more than breastmilk**. Breastfeeding is a relationship, a close physical and emotional relationship between two people who usually love each other. Furthermore, breastfeeding helps to develop that close emotional relationship.

If you cannot produce all the milk the baby needs, you can, and we recommend you do, supplement the baby at the breast with a **lactation aid at the breast**.

Supplements may include formula or donated breastmilk. Please do not pay for donated milk. There are many reported incidents of mothers receiving adulterated breastmilk (usually with formula or cow's milk).

The medications and the process

We generally start the person inducing lactation on a **combination birth control pill** (which provides **both estrogen and progesterone**) as well as **domperidone** which increases prolactin levels.

In theory, **the combination birth control pill** should have higher levels of progesterone, but this is theory, and which combination birth control pill is used probably does not make that much of a difference. If the birth control pill has placebos (that is "sugar pills" or pills without any effect), the person inducing lactation should not take them but rather jump to the next cycle of pills without a break. Remember that during pregnancy the hormonal milieu is not interrupted every month.

The person inducing lactation should be on the combination birth control pill starting as soon as the carrier knows she is pregnant. The person inducing lactation should continue the combination pill until about 6 to 8 weeks before the baby is to be born and then stop the combination pill completely. This implies, usually, about 24 weeks of the combination pill, depending on when the pregnancy is confirmed.

Domperidone increases the prolactin levels in the person inducing lactation and we recommend continuing the domperidone at least until the baby is born and even after that. Indeed, it is likely the domperidone will be needed for the entire period of breastfeeding.

The dose of domperidone? We start with a dose of 30 mg (3 tablets) 3 times a day and sometimes go up from there in two steps, first to 40 mg (4 tablets) 3 times a day and then 40 mg (4 tablets) 4 times a day, or (6 tablets, 5 tablets, 5 tablets, total 16 tablets) since taking medication 3 times a day rather than 4 times a day is more convenient and easier to remember. The main reason not to go to the highest dose immediately is to prevent side effects which may not occur at 9 pills (90 mg/day) but may at 16 pills (160 mg/day).

The side effects of domperidone include weight gain (in about 10% of people taking it), headache, also in about 10%, but which is *usually* mild and transient, lasting no more than a couple of days, and dry mouth. Weight gain also may occur with the birth control pill, and so may headache.

The notion that **domperidone** is dangerous if you have any sort of heart problem is nonsense and is due to formula company disinformation. The only situation where domperidone *might* cause problems is if you have a prolonged QT interval on an electrocardiogram and an electrocardiogram can easily be done to rule out a prolonged QT interval. If you have a heart murmur, if you've had heart surgery, if you have high blood pressure, if you have other findings on electrocardiogram, this is not a reason to avoid domperidone. Our experience with tens of thousands of our patients taking domperidone, is that it is a very safe drug.

Some women may have menstrual irregularities with domperidone, but if they are taking the birth control pill with fairly high levels of estrogen and progesterone, this should not happen. If there is bleeding, she should see her doctor to make sure there is not another source of bleeding.

When the person inducing lactation stops the combination birth control pill, if that person is a woman, she will have a brisk and likely heavy vaginal bleed. This should not last more than a few days.

Once the birth control pill is stopped, the person inducing lactation should start expressing the breasts to stimulate the production of milk. Note that men can produce milk, so that the approach is the same for men. Pumping or expressing the milk should, in theory, be the same as if the baby were breastfed, but in fact, babies vary in their feeding frequency and persons inducing lactation often work outside the home and do not have frequent opportunities to express while at work.

What if I don't have 24 weeks time before the baby is born?

Our preference is not to use the birth control pill and take only the **domperidone**. The problem is that the birth control pill will inhibit milk production, so recommending continuing the birth control pill until after the baby is born, or longer, is not going work well. So, are 14 weeks on the birth control pill plus domperidone okay? Possibly, but it is cutting the time short.

An exception occurs when one of the partners is pregnant and plans to breastfeed and the non-pregnant partner is inducing lactation. In that case, the non-pregnant partner can stay on the birth control pill even after the baby is born to increase the time of her body "thinking it's pregnant", and if the breastfeeding is going well with the pregnant partner, there is no rush to stop the birth control pill.

When do I start putting the baby to the breast?

As soon as possible after the baby's birth. In many jurisdictions the person inducing lactation can take the baby immediately at birth, in the delivery room. In other jurisdictions, this is not possible, but the person inducing lactation should let the hospital staff know in advance that you will be the parent of this baby and that they should avoid feeding the baby with a bottle. A newborn can be fed by spoon or open cup without difficulty.

Should the birth mother feed the baby at the breast?

There are certainly advantages if the birth mother breastfeeds the baby, not only for the baby but also for her. The baby will get the opportunity to receive breastmilk (colostrum) exclusively for a few days or even longer. This also helps the birth mother to **prevent painful engorgement**. Some are happy to breastfeed the baby during the first few days after birth, others not. Others are willing to provide the baby with their milk, but not actually put the baby to the breast. The birth mother may bond with the baby if she feeds the baby to the point where she might not hand over the baby. As far as we know, this has never happened amongst couples attending at our clinic. But the birth mother bonding with the baby is not a bad thing. In fact, it is a good thing.

You and your family doctor

It is important your family doctor know you are taking these medications in case side effects arise. And, it is important s/he know you are inducing lactation, in case side effects of any sort appear and may be related to inducing lactation.

Is it possible to do this without medication?

Some people have not used any of these medications and have just put the baby to the breast. Some have produced milk, even all the milk the baby needed, but this must be a rare situation. Still, if the issue is **breastfeeding and not breastmilk**, this is an option for those people.

RELACTATION

It is possible to start breastfeeding again **even after you have stopped for several weeks or months**

However, first of all, it is important that mothers know that *almost never* is it necessary to stop breastfeeding. Most reasons given for stopping breastfeeding are not valid reasons and most problems resulting in mothers stopping breastfeeding could have been *prevented* or *treated*. Many mothers stop breastfeeding because of some issue, believing that they will simply restart breastfeeding once the issue is sorted out. But stopping breastfeeding for even a few days may result in great difficulties going back to breastfeeding.

Why do mothers feel they must stop or are told they must stop breastfeeding?

• The mother is not producing **enough milk**. Too many health professionals seem to have the idea that some breastmilk is worse than none at all. This is due to the mistaken impression that breastfeeding is necessarily painful or tiring or a burden, or "takes too much out of the mother". This is simply not true, or rather, it *should not be true*. Breastfeeding should be easy, pain free, not tiring, and a pleasure for the mother and the baby. The reason breastfeeding does not always fit this "ideal" picture is due to many reasons, including interventions during labour and birth, especially the large amounts of **intravenous fluids** the mother receives as well as many other **interventions**. As well, after the birth, mothers and babies are subjected to rules about weight loss for which no good evidence exists. Furthermore, the lack of training of hospital staff and physicians with regard to breastfeeding, often results in introduction of **bottles** and **formula** when not necessary, and undermining of the mother's confidence in breastfeeding and making her believe that she is not producing enough milk. Or rather, that the baby is not getting enough milk. A mother can be producing plenty of milk, but the baby may not be getting the milk that is available.

• ʔreastfeeding hurts. Except that breastfeeding should *not* hurt. **Nipple pain** ʔast pain can be prevented and if it occurs, it can often be treated easily, especially if good, skilled help starts early, in the first few days, preferably on the very first day. If breastfeeding hurts, something is not right, and if something is not right it can be fixed. We get referrals to our clinic for mothers having sore nipples for 8 weeks and not infrequently even longer. What is the doctor or midwife thinking? Usually, that "it is normal that breastfeeding hurts, and eventually the pain will stop". And though it is true that sometimes the nipple pain gets better, it's also true that it doesn't always get better. But this sort of thinking results in mothers suffering unnecessarily for weeks and often mothers stopping breastfeeding in desperation. As with all breastfeeding problems, the earlier the mother gets *good* help for sore nipples and breasts, the easier it is to fix the problem.

- The mother is told that the baby needs formula in the first few days postpartum because of **low blood sugar** or because the baby is **jaundiced** or because of **10% weight loss**. The use of bottles may result in the baby not latching on or breastfeeding not becoming well established. Even if supplementation is truly necessary, it should be given **at the breast with a lactation aid**. The lactation aid is not always easy to make work. A baby needs to have a good latch and the tube has to be well placed. Otherwise it is difficult to make work.

- The baby does not latch on. **The main problem with the baby not latching on is the rush to do something, when in fact there is usually no need to rush.** Often when the baby does not latch on, he can be fed by cup or spoon until the mother's milk "comes in". Often, when the milk increases around the third or fourth day, the baby who was not yet latching on, will latch on, especially if the mother has good help available to her. Too often the baby does not latch on because of the early introduction of bottles for dealing with **low blood sugar** or **jaundice** or **10% weight loss**. The most common unnecessary and harmful intervention when the baby is not latching on is for the hospital staff to recommend a **nipple shield**. But for most mothers, all a nipple shield does is *give the impression* that the problem is fixed, when in the long term, and even the short term, the result for most mothers is a **decrease in milk supply**, and subsequent introduction of bottles and, not infrequently, definitive and "permanent" breast refusal.

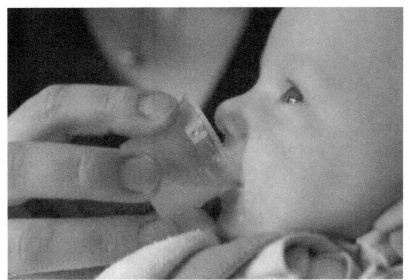

This very few days old baby has not yet latched on. He is being fed expressed breastmilk by cup, which is better than a bottle to feed him and a useful approach to avoid a nipple shield.

- The use of nipple shields is wrongly, but commonly recommended, for **nipple pain**, **breast engorgement**, the baby **not latching on**, and to "teach" a **premature** or even full term baby to breastfeed. This latter reason is even more of an absurdity than the other reasons. All these issues can be solved differently and better without use of a nipple shield. There is nothing that can be done with a nipple shield that cannot be done better without one.

- The mother must take **medication** and is told that she cannot breastfeed while taking this medication. In fact, it is rare that a mother must stop breastfeeding for **medication** she must take.

- A mother with an infection is told that she must not breastfeed because she will pass the infection on to the baby. In fact, the **best protection for the baby** against getting sick in the vast majority of cases is to continue breastfeeding.

- A mother with a non-infectious illness is told that she should not breastfeed because she will need **medication** but the vast majority of medications do not require her to stop breastfeeding. Or she is told she must stop breastfeeding because **breastfeeding is tiring and hard on the mother.** But when breastfeeding is going as it should, most mothers find breastfeeding relaxing, not tiring, pleasant, not a chore.

- The baby has "**breastmilk jaundice**". Too often, the mother is told she must stop breastfeeding when, in fact, it is completely unnecessary and not good for the baby, or the mother for that matter. Even stopping breastfeeding for 2 or 3 days is enough to cause significant breastfeeding problems.

- And there is a host of other reasons, ranging from the absurd to the ridiculous, for which mothers are told they must stop breastfeeding. Or interrupt breastfeeding for various times (for example, some radiological tests, the mother having surgery) and are told that "you can simply just start again" after the "interruption". But, it is simply not true that the mother and baby can simply go back to breastfeeding as it was. After interrupting breastfeeding for even a few days and replacing the baby's feeding with bottles, it can be very difficult to go back to breastfeeding as it was. Even if the mother uses her own milk in the bottle it does not follow that everything will go back to the way it was. The issue is not so much what is in the bottle, but rather, the bottle itself. And don't believe the advertising, there is no bottle that simulates breastfeeding. The result? The frustrated mother then stops breastfeeding.

Thus, the most important step in relactation is to avoid the need to relactate at all, to get good hands on breastfeeding help and advice. Unfortunately, good breastfeeding help is not easily available everywhere.

But you are not breastfeeding any longer. So, what do you do?

The information below is also valid for a mother who is exclusively pumping and would like to have her baby breastfeeding.

There are two points to deal with:

285

1. Getting the baby to take the breast.

2. Increasing/re-establishing the milk supply.

- If the baby is willing to take the breast, **everything is possible**. However, if the baby has not been breastfed for a while, it will probably be necessary to supplement unless your baby is being fed exclusively with your own expressed milk. Even then, the baby, used to bottles, may not latch on well to the breast, resulting in the baby not getting milk well and/or the mother starting to get sore nipples.

- Try to get the **best latch possible**. Know how to know when the baby is **drinking milk from the breast** or **not getting milk from the breast**. If the baby is *not* drinking, only nibbling, try **breast compression** to keep the baby drinking. When the baby is no longer drinking, switch sides and repeat the process. If it is necessary to supplement the baby, it is best done with a **lactation aid at the breast. Domperidone can increase the milk supply.** We start with a dose of 30 mg (3 ten mg tablets) 3 times a day, for a total of 90 mg/day.

- It is best to keep the baby skin to skin as much as possible, with the breast available to the baby. **What is good for premature babies** in terms of skin to skin contact, is good for all babies of any age.

- If the baby is reluctant to take the breast **or completely refuses to take the breast, it is still possible to help the baby latch on. Note that a baby on a nipple shield is not latched on and offering a nipple shield is not an answer.**

- An important step is to stop using bottles and pacifiers. An open cup or a small spoon can be used to feed the baby and these work even in premature babies and are easy to use if the mother is shown how. If the baby is older, say over 3 or 4 months of age, it can be easier to stop the bottles. Instead of feeding the baby by bottle, the baby can be fed **food**, as much as the baby will eat, as frequently as the baby will eat without forcing. Commercial infant cereals are not a good food as they are low in calories and nutrients (except for iron, but most of the iron ends up in the baby's diaper). Many babies this age will eat all

286

sorts of high calorie foods like banana, avocado (30% fat), and foods like mash potatoes without problem. Liquids, preferably breastmilk, butter or oil (vegetable, olive, etc) can be added to the solids.

In this video on www.ibconline.ca, *we see a four month old who has never been exclusively breastfed. This baby does latch on and has continued to latch on because he was always being supplemented with a* **lactation aid at the breast**. *But the mother wanted to stop using the lactation aid. Instead of starting bottles, she could start using an open cup or a small spoon to supplement the baby. But it is possible and preferable to start the baby on* **solids** *as well. So, the baby breastfeeds and eats food – just as any baby would be after about the age of six months. We believe the baby is being offered avocado in this video, but it could be banana.*

- Skin to skin contact with the baby, as much as possible with the bare breast close to the baby. If the breast is available to the baby, the baby may latch on. By increasing the milk supply with **domperidone**, the baby will sense the presence of milk in the breast, the **Montgomery glands of the breast letting the baby know that milk is available**. If the mother can manage to feed breastmilk (by cup, spoon) when skin to skin with the baby and the baby near the breast, this may help the baby to latch on. Taking a bath with the baby, skin to skin, sometimes helps too.

- If nothing is working, the use of **domperidone** and hand expression/pumping will at least get you more milk to feed the baby your breastmilk (used only when you have given the above methods sufficient time and the baby still is just not latching on).

- Be patient. Getting the baby back to breastfeeding may take time but there are many babies who have re-started exclusive breastfeeding after weeks and months of no breastfeeding.

BREASTFEEDING AFTER BREAST SURGERY (PART 1)

As with surgery in any part of the body, surgery on the breast should be undertaken only if necessary and only if other tests (ultrasound, MRI, for example) or treatments have not been helpful in defining or solving the problem. Unfortunately, many surgeons, even some women surgeons, seem to be imbued with an adolescent thinking about breasts; that is, that breasts are for male titillation (sorry) and for sexual purposes only. We do not include all surgeons, of course. Some are sensitive to the principle function of the breast, which is to feed babies and toddlers. But many seem to be completely unaware that the primary reason for the existence of breasts is for feeding babies and toddlers and for comforting and snuggling them. More than one part of the body can have a sexual side as well as another side. The mouth, for example, allows us to eat in order to feed our body and to kiss to show affection.

No other part of the body is looked upon in the same way, where surgery would actually make that part less able to fulfill its function. If a particular surgical technique on the nose, say, resulted in most cases in a person not being able to breathe through the nose, that surgery would be strongly discouraged and even condemned by medical regulatory bodies. But surgery on the breast does not seem to be governed by the same restraint. Once again it may be necessary to repeat that, in affluent societies, breastfeeding is not seen as essential, but, at best, as "nice but not necessary".

We have a video on www.ibconline.ca which shows two mothers breastfeeding. The mother in the first part of the video has had breast reduction surgery. The second part of the video shows another baby drinking extremely well at the breast. Decide whether the first baby is getting enough milk from the breast. You can find the answer at the end of this chapter.

Breast surgery done usually before having babies
(Breast reduction, breast augmentation surgery)

We will not discuss why women might want such surgery, but we think it is fair to say that most, but not all, such surgery is done before a woman has had children. Indeed, if we can judge from our own patients at the International

Breastfeeding Centre, most of the time, the woman having had breast surgery was as young as 14 years old, but more commonly 17 or 18 years old, and has not even dreamed of children in her future yet. And breastfeeding is obviously not part of her thinking. And, in our society, that young woman may not know yet either, like the surgeon, that breasts are for feeding and comforting babies and toddlers.

It is worth knowing that *any* surgery on the breast with an incision done around the areola diminishes the mother's ability to produce milk and therefore should be avoided. The more complete the incision, the more the surgery interferes with milk production. This decrease in the mother's ability to produce milk probably has little to do with the amount of breast tissue that is removed since the decrease also occurs when the periareolar incision is done for a biopsy, for example, where neither a significant amount of breast tissue is removed nor, in other types of surgery, where something (a "prosthesis") is added.

We are making a plea that any surgery on the breast should be made with the purpose of the breast, that is, nourishing babies and toddlers, be always kept in mind. We believe that the vast majority of surgeons never learned how the lactating breast is different from the non-lactating breast and that surgery should be tailored to the function of the breast. Furthermore, even if a young woman is not breastfeeding at the time of surgery, it is possible, even likely, that sometime in the future, she will be breastfeeding, and this too, needs to be considered when operating.

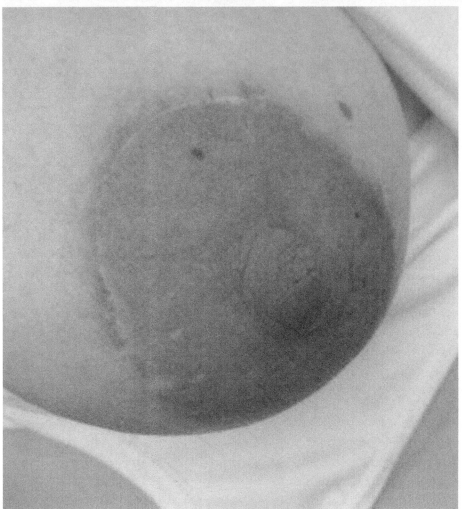

This incision was done for a biopsy of a lump in the breast. It is very long, and the incision follows the line between the areola and the breast. This incision is very likely to interfere with milk production. It is extremely likely that the biopsy could have been done differently.

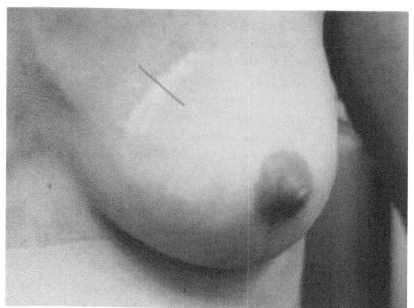

This incision for a breast abscess is more likely to cut several ducts and healing is likely to be delayed as the weight of the breast keeps the incision open. The black line indicates a better incision. It is less likely to cut ducts and the weight of the breast is likely to help heal the incision by keeping the edges close. However, this type of surgery for an abscess is not as good as **catheter drainage**.

In our experience, most women having had breast reduction surgery are unable to produce enough milk, at least with the surgery done with the incision around the areola. Some surgeons have apparently done breast reduction without this type of incision, but we are not aware of any mothers attending our clinic who have had breast reduction surgery done without an incision around the areola. (Liposuction has also been done to decrease the size of the breast, but we have seen only one mother who as this procedure).

Some mothers attending our clinic have been able to breastfeed exclusively after breast reduction, even with complete incisions around the areola, but they are definitely in the minority. However, a few years ago, we did follow one mother who had had breast reduction and, with our help, was able to breastfeed twins exclusively for 6 months and then continued breastfeeding with added **food to the babies' diet**.

When we ask mothers who have had breast reduction surgery what the surgeons told them regarding breastfeeding if they were to go ahead with this type of surgery, the surgeon almost always answered one of two things, both incorrect. Either there would be no problem with breastfeeding, clearly wrong in most cases, or that the chances of breastfeeding are 50%, which, if one thinks about it, makes no sense. In fact, the mother is able to breastfeed. She may have to supplement the baby, preferably with a **lactation aid at the breast**, but she can breastfeed, keeping in mind that **breastfeeding is much more than breastmilk**

What should the surgeon say to the woman asking for breast reduction surgery? That the chances that she will be able to breastfeed her babies *exclusively* are low. And if this woman is 17 or 18 years old, maybe it's better to wait a few years, because the surgery cannot be undone, and perhaps in a couple of years she may have a different outlook on life. And if she decides to have the surgery, then it would be a good idea to get good help and advice about breastfeeding when she is pregnant, so that problems can be avoided as much as possible.

Breast augmentation

If breast augmentation is done with an incision near the chest wall and the prosthesis placed there, no difficulties with breastfeeding seem to occur, at least not from the surgery itself. However, for some reason we can classify only as bizarre, some surgeons do incisions around the areola even for breast augmentation. If the incision is around the areola, then milk production will be compromised just as it is with breast reduction. There can be only two reasons that we can understand for doing an incision around the areola for breast augmentation. Either the surgeon does not know this may negatively affect breastfeeding, and if this is the case, then how can the surgeon be operating on a gland s/he does not know anything about? Or, the surgeon does not care that breastfeeding will be negatively impacted. Basically, "breastfeeding is nice, but not necessary".

SOLUTION to the video: The first baby shown in the video is getting a fair amount of milk from the breast, but the baby drank even less well on the other breast (not shown in the video). As a result, the total intake of breastmilk was less milk than the baby required, and as a result, the mother needed to supplement the baby, with a **lactation aid at the breast** (production of milk from both breasts is frequently very unequal after breast reduction, which is sometimes even if the mother has not had breast surgery). You can learn how to tell whether a baby is getting milk from the breast or not by **watching more of our videos** and reading the explanatory texts which discuss the pause in the chin.

Continue reading about **surgery done on the breast at a time when the mother is breastfeeding** a baby and **when she finds a lump in her breast**.

BREAST SURGERY AND ITS EFFECT ON BREASTFEEDING (PART 2)

There are **surgeries that are done on the breasts before a woman has children** and can impact her ability to produce milk. This chapter discusses surgery on the lactating breast.

Galactocoeles and breast abscess

Blebs/blocked ducts/mastitis and on occasion, abscess, usually occur when the mother has an abundant milk supply, but the baby does not have a good latch. A galactocoele seems to arise in a blocked duct if the blocked duct does not resolve quickly.

And why does the baby not latch on well?

Because of

- How the baby is positioned and latched on.

- **The use of artificial nipples** such as bottles, and **nipple shields**, and more than occasional use of pacifiers.

- The baby has a tongue tie. Some tongue ties are obvious, but many tongue ties are more subtle and require an evaluation that goes farther than just looking but includes feeling under the baby's tongue, evaluating the upward mobility of the tongue, as well and knowing what is normal and not normal. The truth is, however, that few health professionals, including many lactation consultants, know how to evaluate whether or not the baby has a tongue tie.

- The mother has had a decrease in her milk supply. On the other hand, blebs/blocked ducts/mastitis may also occur because milk supply has *decreased*. Recurrent blocked ducts and sometimes even a single blocked duct or mastitis may result in milk supply decreasing. **Late onset decreased milk supply** is common in our clinic experience, and results the baby slipping down

294

on the nipple and pulling at the breast. The baby may pull off the breast when milk flow slows resulting in a breast that does not drain well. In fact, the mother may feel her milk supply is still good, even "overabundant" because the breasts are frequently "full", even immediately after a feeding. Watch our videos on www.ibconline.ca: **Really good drinking with English text, Twelve day old nibbling, English Text, "Borderline" drinking** for video clips showing babies drinking well at the breast, or not. Watch the videos, read the texts and then watch the videos again. Following the **Protocol to manage BM intake** may change things so the baby does gain well.

Galactocoele or milk cyst

We make the diagnosis of a galactocoele by aspirating milk from the fluid filled lump in the breast. Neither history nor physical examination and often not even ultrasound examination are reliable ways of knowing if the lump is a galactocoele or something else. If the aspiration yields milk, the lump is a galactocoele. If it yields pus, it is an abscess. Once the diagnosis is made (by aspiration), we believe the best thing to do with a galactocoele is to *leave it alone.*

True, when palpating the lump, one usually gets the impression that there is fluid in the lump, but not always, especially if the galactocoele or abscess are relatively deep in the breast. Also, the feeling of fluid in the lump does not distinguish a galactocoele from an abscess. An abscess tends to be tender if squeezed, but not particularly painful unless rapidly enlarging. A galactocoele is usually not tender and not painful unless rapidly enlarging.

Once the diagnosis is proved, yes, we are repeating ourselves in order to emphasize that a galactocoele should be left alone. Repeated aspirations of a galactocoele do nothing as the galactocoele will quickly refill after aspiration. Though the risk of infection is low if aspiration is properly done, each aspiration does carry a small risk of infection. A galactocoele can be quite large but usually stops growing once the pressure inside the galactocoele equals the pressure outside the galactocoele.

Doing surgery on a galactocoele as recommended by some surgeons is a recipe for disaster especially since it is rarely necessary. A galactocoele will disappear once the mother stops breastfeeding, but she should not stop breastfeeding simply because the galactocoele is there. It causes no harm in the long run to leave it alone.

This photo shows what can go wrong when a galactocoele is operated upon. True, the result is rarely this bad, but this sort of result is not okay even if it does occur only rarely.

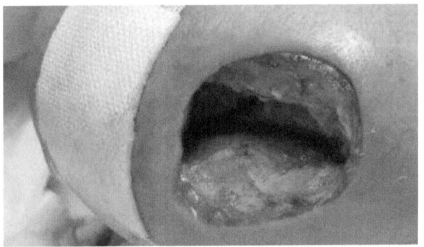

This mother had surgery for a galactocoele (milk cyst). It is rarely, if ever, necessary to do surgery on a milk cyst. This is a disastrous result.

Less dramatic but also a problem is that the mother will have continued leaking of milk from the incision after the surgery. In effect, the galactocoele has been "exteriorized". Instead of the milk staying inside the breast, the milk now leaks out (sometimes pours) into the mother's clothing. And the leaking is more likely if, as usual, the mother is told by the surgeon to stop breastfeeding on that side (or stop completely). Where will the milk go out, if it doesn't go out the usual way, through the nipple? Out the area of least resistance to the flow of fluid, the incision. So, it is best that the mother continue breastfeeding and the milk "exits" the usual way.

If the mother in the photo above had not had surgery, she would have remained with a lump in the breast, unlikely to be more than mildly painful, and she would have continued breastfeeding. The galactocoele would most likely have dried up once she stopped breastfeeding. As it is, she was hospitalized for the procedure and stayed in hospital for well over a week. And even then, her problems were not over.

Breast abscess

The history of breast abscess frequently follows a typical time line. A mother develops the signs and symptoms of mastitis, sees her physician and is treated with an **antibiotic, often an inappropriate one**. Even though it has been known for years that the most common infecting organism in mastitis, by far, is *Staphylococcus aureus*, too often mothers are treated with antibiotics such as amoxicillin or erythromycin. Amoxicillin will not kill *Staphylococcus aureus* and only a small minority of *Staphylococcus aureus* is sensitive to erythromycin. Furthermore, the nausea, vomiting and abdominal pain that occurs not infrequently with erythromycin make it a poor choice for treating mastitis.

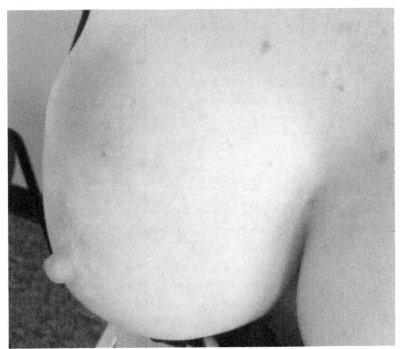

Typical presentation of a breast abscess. Redness is common but not universal; a lump is easily felt in the breast and is painful when squeezed; there is a history of mastitis treated inappropriately.

Even worse, many mothers are told they must stop breastfeeding when they have mastitis or when **taking antibiotics**. This makes no sense at all, and it should be pointed out that a time-honoured principle of medical and surgical treatment is to encourage drainage of an area of infection and swelling. And the best way to do that is to have the baby continue to breastfeed on the affected side.

Furthermore, the concern about the baby getting the infection is not valid. First of all, the mother had the bacteria on her body well before developing the mastitis and so the baby has been exposed to the bacteria well before the mother was aware of being unwell. In fact, breastfeeding mothers and babies share all their germs, and this is a good thing. **Furthermore, breastfeeding protects babies against infection**; this has been known for years, but it seems many modern doctors have forgotten, even though the evidence continues to accumulate of how protective breastfeeding is.

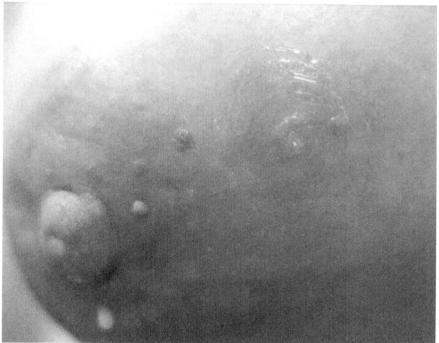

An abscess may drain on its own. In this case, the abscess has neared the skin and is about to burst through the skin . Note that the mother's milk looks normal, there is no pus in the milk. If there were a connection between the abscess and the milk ducts, the abscess would "cure itself" by draining.

As for the mother taking antibiotics, **this is not a reason to interrupt breastfeeding**. The antibiotics used for the treatment of mastitis are also drugs we use frequently for babies should they require them (and too often when they *don't* require them, but that's another story). The amount of any drug that enters the milk is minuscule and antibiotics are not exceptions.

What to do

The first thing to emphasize is that a breast abscess, though distressing to the mother and the physician, is not a dire emergency. Mothers and babies are too frequently sent rushing to the emergency department for immediate treatment when a more restrained, thoughtful approach would be much better.

The diagnosis of breast abscess can be made by aspirating the mass (photo below). This not only makes the diagnosis (aspiration will reveal that the content of the mass is pus) but also gives some relief to the mother if she is in pain. Furthermore, a sample for the laboratory for culture and sensitivity of the organism causing the abscess is available (almost always, in our experience, *Staphylococcus aureus* and not rarely these days MRSA – methicillin resistant *Staphylococcus aureus*).

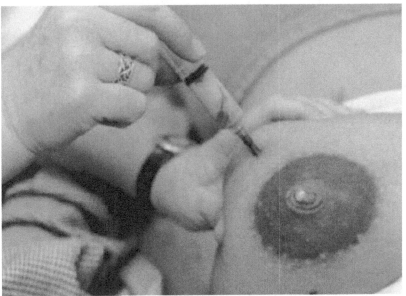

Making the diagnosis of breast abscess is by aspirating the contents of the lump in the breast. Again, the milk does not contain pus.

Aspirations can be repeated every few days if necessary, but this routine of returning to the doctor's office over and over is not easy for a new mother and her baby and even less so if she has other young children at home.

Furthermore, repeated aspirations do not always work to treat the abscess definitively.

However, incision and drainage, as done by most surgeons also is not a good idea. Surgeons, *as a group*, (of course there are exceptions), do not seem to consider breastfeeding important. Stopping breastfeeding on the affected breast, which, at least from our experience, most surgeons recommend, risks milk continuing to leak out the incision once the infection is cured, as with a galactocoele. Where will the milk come out if not from the nipple? Yes, the area of least resistance, the incision. And not emptying the breast by breastfeeding causes the mother additional pain from engorgement.

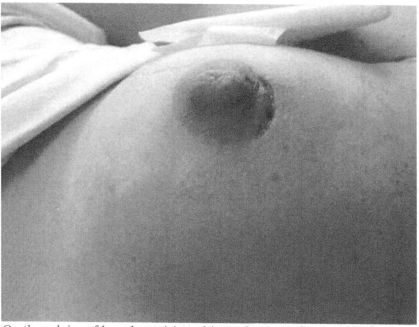

*On the advice of her obstetrician, this mother specifically asked the surgeon not to do an incision around the areola and yet he did it anyway. Furthermore, the surgery was done under general anaesthesia, which is not necessary with the **procedure recommended below**. How will the mother be able to put the baby to this breast after the surgery? The incision is exactly where the baby would need to latch on. Every principle of treating a breast abscess in a breastfeeding mother has been violated in this case. This type of*

incision not only diminishes the mother's milk supply for this baby but also for every baby from now on.

Some surgeons go even further and strongly recommend the mother stop breastfeeding completely, even on the unaffected side. Now why would they do this?

The reason, I think, is that they want the breast with the abscess to dry up (well, why the breast with the abscess needs to dry up is another question). And surgeons, *as a group*, do not seem to understand that a mother can dry up on just one breast *if it is necessary*, which it usually is not. They believe, it seems, that breastfeeding on the unaffected breast will keep the milk going on the affected side, the one with the abscess. Do they really understand so little about breastfeeding and how the breastfeeding works? What would we think about a gastrointestinal surgeon who didn't understand how the gut works?

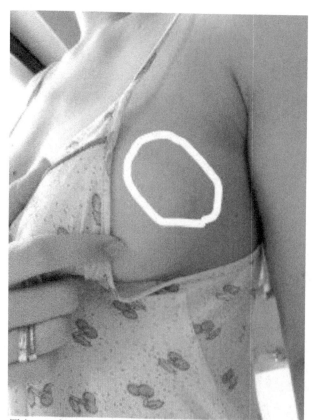

This mother had a breast abscess drained by surgery. The scar (indicated by white circle) shows the incision was very large. The mother was told she would have to stop breastfeeding on this side to prevent prolonged leaking from the incision (a fistula). I suggested she should not interrupt breastfeeding. It took a month for the incision to close and it did close even though the mother continued to breastfeed on this side.

The way to treat an abscess?

If we diagnose a breast abscess, we will send the mother and baby to an intervention radiologist who uses another approach than incision and drainage favoured by the surgeon. This approach allows the baby to continue breastfeeding on both breasts while resulting in far fewer complications for the mother. The approach is outlined in **this article**.

Here's how it works: The radiologist maps out the abscess with ultrasound and inserts a catheter into the abscess to drain it. The catheter is kept in place until there is no further drainage and then removed. The mother continues breastfeeding on the affected side as she would have normally if she hadn't developed the abscess.

In general, we continue antibiotics based on the sensitivity of the bacterium until the mother is cured.

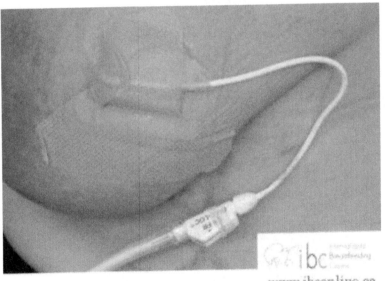

www.ibconline.ca

Catheter placed into abscess cavity after mapping out the abscess by ultrasound. Note that the mother can still breastfeed as there is no incision near the areola and no dressing impeding latching on. This mother's abscess was cured with this procedure.

Our experience with this procedure?

In the 12 or more years that we have been referring our patients with breast abscess to the intervention radiologists at the nearby hospital, we have seen a few more than 100 mothers with a breast abscess. Happily, the numbers have decreased over the years. One can hope that this is because fewer mothers are developing an abscess due to their getting better help with positioning and latching babies on, as well as other rational information on breastfeeding, but I wonder. Perhaps more mothers are being referred to intervention radiologists rather than to surgeons.

So what results have we had? Only one mother that I can remember stopped breastfeeding despite our encouragement to keep breastfeeding. One mother had a recurrence of an abscess which was treated in the same way and she she was then cured. One mother, we feared, was developing a fistula (a leakage of milk from the site of the catheter insertion that does not stop), but in fact, after 3 weeks the leakage stopped on its own. All the rest of the mothers were cured with this procedure without stopping breastfeeding on the affected breast.

Does incision and drainage, the surgeon's approach, prevent recurrence? No, according to the literature about 7% of abscesses recur after incision and drainage. As you can see, our results show a rate of recurrence of less than 1%.

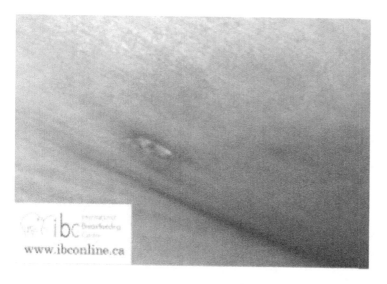

www.ibconline.ca

One week after removal of the catheter (not the same mother as figure 5). Total time from drainage of the abscess? About 2 weeks

Continue reading about **what to do in case you find a lump in your breast** at a time when you are breastfeeding your baby.

BREAST SURGERY AND BREASTFEEDING (PART 3)

EVALUATION OF A BREAST LUMP

This chapter is part 3 of 3 chapters, the first two of which discuss breast surgery done on the breast before the mother has a baby and breast surgery done on the breast at a time when the mother is breastfeeding.

When a breastfeeding mother or her physician finds a lump in the breast, the question of what to do arises. In breastfeeding mothers, the most common reasons for a lump in the breast would likely be the following:

–A blocked duct (which tends to resolve quickly and often without specific treatment)
–Mastitis (which also frequently resolves without specific treatment)
–Abscess (which often opens spontaneously to the skin and thus is often cured without specific treatment)
–Galactocele (which usually should be left alone once the diagnosis is made)

–And all sorts of benign lumps not related to breastfeeding, which may include a fibroadenoma, benign cysts, papilloma, fat necrosis, hamartomas.

Unfortunately, it is also possible for a mother to develop breast cancer while breastfeeding.

Here is a not uncommon situation as described by a breastfeeding mother:

"Two lumps were found in my breast during my pregnancy, and it was recommended I get them biopsied. I got the core biopsy done at ten days postpartum. I have had constant milk leakage from the incision site (6 days now). Yesterday I soaked through 4 hospital maxi pads. I went to the doctor today and was told that the lumps were benign fibroadenomas, and to wait 1 week to see if the leaking stops, and if it doesn't, I'll need to stop breastfeeding altogether. She said if I wait longer, I'm at high risk for infection & mastitis. I don't want to stop breastfeeding, and I'm wondering how often milk duct fistulas heal on their own. Just want your opinion and what you recommend."

The first question that arises is why it was necessary to go to biopsy before other diagnostic methods were tried first. Imaging methods have improved considerably over the past few years and continue to improve, and their judicious use can avoid the need for biopsy in many, but not all, cases. An ultrasound done even during the pregnancy could have helped allay the mother's worries, although it is unlikely one can get a definite diagnosis from an ultrasound. A CT scan or MRI scan could have given enough information to avoid the biopsy. Positron Emission Tomography (PET scan) can also be done to characterize a breast lump in certain circumstances, though it does not seem to be commonly used for characterizing breast lumps and should not be done during pregnancy.

A mammogram is not ideal for a breastfeeding mother because of the compression of the breast while the procedure is done. Mammograms have been traditionally used for screening but alone, they do not really help often in diagnosing a breast lump.

Finally, one must ask the question: if it was necessary to do a biopsy, why was the biopsy not done during the pregnancy when the risks of complications would be far less?

It is necessary to emphasize that neither **CT scan, nor MRI require the mother to interrupt breastfeeding**, not even for a minute. See the bulletins from the **American College of Radiology** and **Society of Urogenital Radiology** which have both issued statements in 2001 and 2004 respectively stating that a breastfeeding mother can continue breastfeeding after these tests without any interruption at all. **My article** discusses the same question. With PET scan, with the half-life of the isotope being less than 2 hours, it is recommended that close contact between mother and baby be avoided for 4 hours after the procedure.

We are not saying that biopsy is never required to characterize a breast lump. However, if appropriate, a fine needle biopsy is less likely to cause continued leaking (fistula) from the biopsy site than a core biopsy, which uses a larger needle, and core biopsy is less likely to cause a fistula than an open biopsy.

Ultimately, a decision of how to investigate a breast lump in a breastfeeding mother has to take into consideration which approach results in the best way of diagnosing the breast lump without interfering with the mother's ability to continue breastfeeding. If the lump is unlikely to be cancerous, less aggressive methods should be tried first. If it is very likely to be cancerous, then a more aggressive approach would be necessary. However, in the case above, it is unlikely that the lump was considered very likely to be cancerous, or the mother would have been advised to have diagnosis made during the pregnancy. Indeed, a core biopsy would have caused far fewer problems during the pregnancy than a core biopsy during lactation.

Incorrect information described in the mother's story

This mother was told that there was a risk of infection or mastitis if the leaking did not stop. This is not true. Why would this occur if the milk is free flowing out the biopsy site?

And it makes no sense to say that if after another week the leaking hadn't stopped, the mother would have to stop breastfeeding completely. What's wrong with this advice?

1. It sounds as if the mother was told not to breastfeed on the side of the biopsy, though this is not 100% clear from the email. Stopping on the affected side increases the risk of a fistula because if the milk doesn't go out the nipple, it will go out where it can go out, the area of least resistance, the incision.

2. The time line of 1 week (after 6 days after the biopsy) for the leaking to stop or the mother must stop breastfeeding is very short. Why 1 week? What if the leaking is decreasing but not stopped? We have seen leaking for 2 or 3 weeks after such procedures and the leaking does stop even when the mother continues breastfeeding on the affected side.

3. Many surgeons do not seem to understand that it is possible to stop breastfeeding on one side while continuing on the other if that becomes truly necessary. This is the reason for the mother being told to stop breastfeeding completely. But if worse gets to worst, the mother could stop on just the affected side. Eventually, the leaking will stop.

TO SLEEP, PERCHANCE TO DREAM

It is the dream of every parent of young babies and toddlers to get some sleep. Endless longing to be able to sleep influences how people feel about breastfeeding since they attribute much of their lack of sleep to breastfeeding.

"Sleep issues" are among the top reasons for supplementing with formula or even stopping breastfeeding completely even when everything else is going well with breastfeeding:

- Many parents give their babies a bottle of formula to get them to sleep at night.
- Getting the baby to "sleep through the night" is seen as a reason for "night weaning" of the baby or for stopping breastfeeding altogether.
- Some parents "top up" with formula after a breastfeed to get the baby to fall asleep.
- Some fathers or other family members bottle feed their otherwise breastfed babies at night so that the breastfeeding mother may get some sleep.
- Some psychologists/psychiatrists, in order to prevent postpartum depression have thought it wise for the baby to be fed formula by bottle in the night, by someone other than the mother, so that the mother will be able to sleep though the night.
- Some parents worry that the baby is not getting enough milk in case the baby does not fall asleep once they have breastfed.
- How long a baby sleeps is sometimes taken as a measure of whether the baby received enough breastmilk or not and if the baby wakes up after a 20 or 40 minute nap, it is taken as a sign of "low milk supply".

Breastfeeding and sleep are inextricably connected. So much so that James McKenna describes the interconnectedness of the two as "breastsleeping" – i.e. sleeping by breastfeeding and breastfeeding while sleeping.

People are really losing their sleep over the erroneous notions around baby sleep that have been created in the past 100 years; erroneous notions based on the formula fed baby as the "model" for baby behaviour. They, and health professionals, have forgotten how babies sleep and what is normal. They have accepted that there is only one correct way to sleep for both babies and adults

– 8 hours of uninterrupted sleep. And everyone who does not sleep that way has a "sleep problem". People have come to believe that they can "turn babies off", like the light, for the night. Consequently, the baby sleeping through the night has become many parents' life goal supported by hosts of "baby sleep trainers" who promote various versions of controlled crying or crying it out "solutions".

In fact, sleeping 8 hours in a row was not considered **normal even for adults until fairly recently.** References from as long ago as Homer's time (not Homer Simpson, Homer the Greek poet) to the 17th century describe a first sleep which began about two hours after dusk, followed by waking period of one or two hours and then a second sleep.

Contrary to people's endless search for the Eldorado of parenting – sleeping through the night as soon as possible – James McKenna explains that waking up at night while "breastsleeping" is good for the baby because it provides protection to the baby because:

- the baby gets to be checked
- the baby absorbs all sorts of stimuli from the mother such as her breathing out carbon dioxide which helps the baby to breathe more continuously
- the baby absorbs also her smell, her touch, her warmth, the movement of her chest
- the baby spends the night in safer *lighter* sleep
- the baby gets to practice getting awake quickly which is important in SIDS prevention
- the baby grows specific brain architecture
- and the baby's lighter sleep terminates apneas (abnormal cessation of breathing, said to be more than 20 seconds) which occur during too deep sleep.

In other words, it is far more important for a baby's health and survival to learn to sleep *lightly* and to awaken quickly, than to learn to sleep deeply without waking up. "Sensory deprivation" and "arousal deficiency" is what happens to babies who are missing the stimulation the mother's body provides.

In a laboratory study, mothers experienced 30% more arousals when they slept with their infants (Mosko et al 1997a). And mother-infant pairs tended to sleep in synchrony, with more than 70% of their arousals overlapping (Mosko et al 1997b). Moreover, mothers who bed-shared checked on their babies more frequently during the night. In **Baddock's study**, bed sharing mothers checked on their babies a median of 11 times. For mothers sleeping in separate beds, the median was 4 times.

Knowing all this and accepting how babies sleep goes a long way to sleeping better at night because much of the sleeplessness parents experience is caused by their endless struggle to "create good sleeping habits". And what really keeps parents awake at night is worrying that there is something intrinsically wrong with their baby or toddler who keeps waking up at night.

The myth of "sleeping through the night" is preventing us from asking the most essential question: "What sort of sleeping arrangement makes babies feel best?" It is not in the baby's best interest to sleep deeply and through the night.

Throughout pregnancy the baby's existence and well-being are conditional on his being regulated by his mother's body – the baby is in constant physical contact with the mother, receives sensory input from his mother, is rocked to sleep by his mother and is awake when his mother is motionless. It is an exercise in futility to act on the notion that babies lose the need for all this sensory input and physical contact as soon as they are born and that their desire to be constantly close to their mothers is a result of being spoiled and is a bad habit. It is remarkable how much independence is being required of newborns or 4 month old babies. "Sleeping through the night" and "babies self-soothing and being independent" were two concepts that appeared as a direct result of the wide spread use of formula which enabled both daytime and nighttime separation of mothers and babies. But biology does not change as fast as culture.

Additionally, parents have been made to feel guilty for letting their baby fall asleep at the breast once they have breastfed well because they were led to believe that babies should be taught to fall asleep on their own and to "self-soothe". Breastfeeding, however, has, as one of its functions to put both the mother and baby to sleep.

It is normal for mothers to feel drowsy towards the end of the feeding and it is normal for babies to fall asleep at the breast. Many parents get frustrated when they spend their time trying to "break" this sleep association. In many languages of the world the word breastfeeding translates as "calming down" or "quiet down" – all references to what breastfeeding does for the baby in order to enable his transition from being awake to being sleepy to falling asleep.

The need to suck in order to fall asleep is obvious to parents – that is why so many use pacifiers as a substitute for the breast. This has actually reached absurd proportions when people turn the physiological function of breastsleeping around and say, "The baby is using me as a pacifier." In fact, the breastsleeping baby is only doing what his innate physiology is telling him to do – falling asleep by breastfeeding.

In order for breastfeeding and sleeping to work together the first step is to ensure the baby is breastfeeding well and getting enough milk from the breast. How?

- Ensure the baby has the **best latch possible**. This is most important in the first days and weeks, and after that, the baby "gets it" and does it on his own, as long as he doesn't receive bottles and pacifiers. Or is feeding on a **nipple shield**.
- Learn how you can tell whether the baby is getting milk from the breast or not by watching these videos on www.ibconline.ca: **Really good drinking with English text, Twelve day old nibbling, English Text, "Borderline" drinking** for video clips showing babies drinking well at the breast, or not or somewhere in between.
- Learn how to use **breast compressions** to increase the amount of breastmilk the baby gets.
- Switch sides when the baby is no longer drinking even with compressions.
- If you are unsure whether your baby is getting enough and/or you have sore nipples, and/or a baby who does not gain weight, and/or is fussy, and/or crying, and/or "colicky", and/or your baby is not exclusively breastfed, and/or does not latch on well or has other issues, make an **appointment at our clinic**

or see someone who knows how to provide practical hands on help with breastfeeding.

What if your baby or toddler is thriving and breastfeeding well...

... and yet you are unsure about what do to about your baby's sleep, here are some tips:

Your baby needs help to fall asleep. Expecting the baby to "self-soothe" and magically fall asleep on his own leads to a lot of crying while parents are hoping the baby will somehow understand that he should fall asleep. Thus, it is important that you find a way to help your baby fall asleep. What can you do?

- Let your baby fall asleep at the breast once he has breastfed well. The baby will usually gently release the breast as he falls asleep.

- Take your baby to bed, breastfeed the baby while lying down and let him fall asleep.

- Wait until your baby is really asleep (this may take much longer than you expect) and do not put the baby down before he is asleep.

- Walk your baby to sleep by putting him in a carrier or a wrap while breastfeeding him at the same time. Or take him for a walk as he feeds.

- Put your baby to sleep before he is too tired and overstimulated.

- Vertical motion (up and down) helps babies to quiet down and fall asleep. One way to do this is to use a big exercise ball to gently rock the baby up and down.

- Know that falling asleep gets easier and easier for babies as they grow older.

- Make sure your baby gets enough sleep. Some parents try to have their babies sleep as little as possible during the day hoping the baby will sleep better at night. However, for babies it is important to get good sleep both during the day and at night. In any case, trying to keep the baby up longer during the day so he will sleep longer at night hardly ever works, if ever. Just as breastfeeding and sleeping are interconnected, so is sleep and brain development. Lighter sleep and frequent night-time waking are connected to memory formation and developing brain.

- Use skin to skin contact to help your baby calm down and fall asleep.

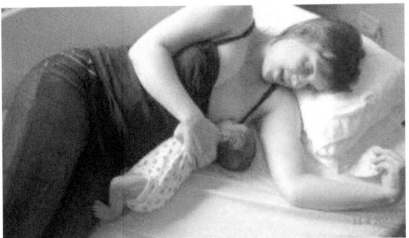

This mother is feeding her baby lying down, side by side with her baby. Well-latched on babies often seem to get more milk when they are feeding side by side with the mother as in the photo. This works particularly well when the mother has less milk, as in the evening. Generally, babies seem calmer in this position particularly in the evening.

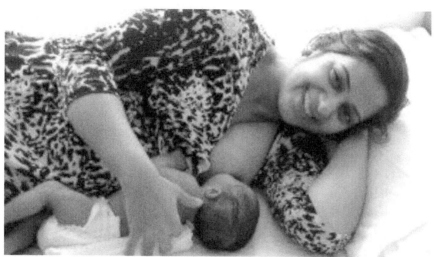

Lying side by side and feeding the baby is a good way for the mother to rest and to sleep together with the baby.

Formula marketing tries to convince us that formula is the answer to "sleep problems". Formula companies make all sorts of "good night" and "good sleep" formulas and this leads to some people giving babies formula just to put their baby to sleep or to get the baby to fall asleep during night.

Instead of giving babies a bottle of formula at night, make sure the baby is breastfeeding well and increase your milk supply if necessary. Often mothers observe that they have more milk in the morning and early afternoon and less in the late afternoon and evening and that their babies are more difficult to put to sleep in the evening. The answer may be increasing milk supply. If your baby is breastfeeding well, then developing strategies to help the baby relax and fall asleep is what is necessary.

However unbelievable it may sound, babies will eventually sleep through the night and there is no reason for "night weaning" in order to achieve that. Nighttime breastfeeding provides security to the baby as well as transition from one sleep cycle to the next. Statistically speaking, the overall length of breastfeeding is heavily dependent on the baby and toddler breastfeeding at

317

night. There are other things you can do to help you feel better about the night during which your baby wakes up frequently to breastfeed:

- Accepting the situation goes a long way.

- Taking your baby to bed with you.

- Making sure you have enough comfortable sleeping space. Feeling cramped in a too small bed or worrying that the baby might fall out of bed can cause you to sleep less well than you would. Putting a mattress on the floor and sleeping there with the baby may help a lot.

- Knowing that you are helping your baby's physiology to receive the stimuli he needs for the right sleep cycling and brain development can help you accept the situation as well.

- Stopping counting the times your baby woke up at night. If you avoid the counting, "nighttime harmony" will develop in which you wake up a few seconds before your baby, put him to the breast and continue sleeping without almost noticing the interruption. Nighttime harmony is disrupted if the baby is getting bottles from other members of the family who might be hoping to help you by "letting you sleep while they give the baby a bottle". In the long run, giving bottles to the baby at night may lower your milk production too because some babies get a lot of their breastmilk intake at night and milk production is to some extent connected with breastfeeding at night – sleeping with your baby at night increases the number of times the baby breastfeeds and because most babies breastfeed well at night and get plenty of milk, it increases mothers' milk supply.

- Starting breastfeeding your baby as soon as your baby stirs instead of waiting for full blown crying which may make the baby inconsolable.

- Knowing that the average sleep cycle of a baby at night is about 90 minutes.

- Trying to go to sleep as soon as the baby goes to sleep at night instead of using the first sleep of the baby to stay up.

Rest assured that eventually all babies will sleep through the night and begin to fall asleep on their own as well and it can be done without letting them cry it out. They simply "grow up" and what changes is how long it takes for them to fall asleep and their sleep patterns naturally change. They begin to transition from sleep cycle to the next without needing the help of breastfeeding.

HOW WHAT IS GOOD ABOUT BREASTFEEDING IS MADE BAD (PART 1)

Many physicians as well as anti-breastfeeding activists manage to turn logic on its head and push the notion that what is good about breastfeeding is, in fact, bad for the mother or baby. Two examples follow.

1. Breastmilk contains antibodies that protect the baby against infection

Unlike what many people, including many physicians, think, breastmilk has *many* diverse immune factors, not only antibodies, that help to protect the baby against infection. The fact that even exclusively breastfed babies sometimes get infections often is taken as "proof" that breastmilk does not really offer much protection in "first world societies". That, of course, proves nothing at all, since no measure of protection is perfect. And, it should not be forgotten that while breastfed babies are *actively* protected, formula fed babies in affluent societies are protected because they are generally "cloistered", kept away from all possible sources of infection. A hopeless stratagem actually.

However, the formula "pushers" forget that we have our own "third world" even within some of the wealthiest countries of the world; in the slums of the cities, in some areas of the countryside, and in the First Nations reserves, in Canada and the US.

Breastmilk contains many immune factors, dozens in fact, working together, helping to protect the baby against infection. As mentioned above, antibodies represent just one of these factors.

One important way, but not the only way, breastmilk actively protects the baby is by forming a barrier of immune factors on the linings of the digestive tract and respiratory tract that blocks bacteria, viruses and fungi from entering the baby's body (anything inside the digestive tract or respiratory tract is considered outside the body). The vast majority of antibodies in the milk are called sIgA ("secretory" IgA, made up of two molecules of the antibody IgA, with an added secretory chain which allows the molecule to get into the milk and a J chain which protects the molecule from digestion by gastric and intestinal

320

enzymes). The sIgA molecules make up part of this protective barrier, but the barrier is made up of lactoferrin, lysozyme, mucins and other immune factors; however, the sIgA antibodies do not get absorbed into the baby's bloodstream. Some people who do not know what they are talking about have said (and even written in books) that the antibodies can protect the baby only against gut infections (gastroenteritis) because the antibodies don't get into the baby's bloodstream. But obviously they don't know how this barrier works. Clearly, it is better to prevent the bacteria, viruses and fungi from getting into the baby's body in the first place rather than fight them off once they have invaded into the baby.

Mothers with autoimmune diseases are often told they cannot breastfeed

Many mothers who have conditions caused by antibodies against their own tissues (Graves' disease, Hashimoto thyroiditis, lupus erythematosus, idiopathic thrombocytopenic purpura, autoimmune hemolytic anemia, rheumatoid arthritis and others) are told that they should not breastfeed because the antibodies causing their disease will get into the milk and cause the same disease in the baby.

This is simply not true. First of all, the sIgA, which is the main antibody in breastmilk, making up at least 95% of all the antibodies in the milk, does not get absorbed from the baby's gut, so it cannot get into the baby's body and cause disease. Secondly, the antibodies that cause these diseases such as rheumatoid arthritis are not of the IgA type and, in any case, they would not get into the milk in any but insignificant amounts. Even if they did, they would be destroyed in the baby's stomach (sIgA does not get destroyed because it has that J chain which protects it from digestive enzymes). And even if the antibodies causing autoimmune diseases somehow did get past the digestive enzymes, they also would not be absorbed into the baby's body.

So, if the mother has a condition in which antibodies in her body attack her own tissues, the mother can and should breastfeed her baby with confidence that she is doing the best for her baby and not worry about the antibodies getting into the milk and causing a problem for the baby.

321

But the baby could be born with the same problem!

True, in conditions such as those mentioned above, the baby is often born with the same problem as the mother due to antibodies passing over to the baby through the placenta. For example, a baby whose mother has idiopathic thrombocytopenia purpura (where the mother has low platelets caused by antibodies against platelets, thus causing them to be destroyed) will often be born with low platelets as well, since the mother's antibodies passed *through the placenta* to the baby during the pregnancy, but **not from the milk**. This effect on the baby is obvious because the platelet count is easy to measure, a routine part of the blood count along with hemoglobin, hematocrit and white blood cell counts. The baby's low platelet count can be present for a few weeks after birth, but only rarely is the platelet count so low as to cause a real risk of bleeding. With time, usually by six or eight weeks after the baby's birth, the platelet count of the baby will be rising since the antibodies will be disappearing from his blood.

Another situation in which the problem is easy to measure occurs when the mother has autoimmune hemolytic anemia, a condition due to antibodies against the mother's red blood cells, resulting in anemia. The baby can be born with his red blood cell count low because of the antibodies that passed into his body *during the pregnancy*. Both idiopathic thrombocytopenic purpura and autoimmune hemolytic anemia almost always improve without specific treatment unless the baby's platelets, in the one case, or the red blood cells, in the other, are very low and require transfusion, which is only rarely necessary.

Yet another situation occurs when the mother has Graves' disease which causes hyperthyroidism (overactive thyroid). The antibodies in the mother's blood *cross the placenta*, as with the other conditions discussed above and the baby is born with signs of hyperthyroidism; rapid heart rate (over 160/minute), jitteriness, high blood pressure and even congestive heart failure if severe. Poor weight gain may also occur. Treatment of the baby's symptoms is possible with drugs that block the effect of the overactive thyroid. But again, there is no reason to restrict breastfeeding.

In *rare* cases, however, the baby continues to have the above problems much longer than the usual 6 to 8 weeks. It seems very *unlikely* that this is due to the continued presence of antibodies from the pregnancy which disappear from the baby's blood within the first few weeks at most, and as mentioned above, impossible to explain as being due to antibodies in the milk. More likely, there are cytokines, small proteins that can affect immune responsiveness in the baby and result in continued problems.

A prolonged effect on the blood cells or platelets as well as other such syndromes, longer, say, than two to three months is unusual, even rare, and no reason to tell the mother not to breastfeed from birth as is often done. Should prolonged low platelets or low hemoglobin or other syndromes occur, longer than 3 or 4 months, despite treatment such as transfusion or oral corticosteroids in the baby, stopping breastfeeding may be considered. It should be pointed out that low platelets, unless severe, are not usually associated with a high risk of bleeding.

Breastmilk varies from woman to woman, **from the beginning of the feeding to the end of the feeding, from morning until night, according to what the mother might have eaten, from early in lactation (colostrum), to later in lactation. In other words, the milk changes according to the needs of the child. Because of this, some people begin to have some strange ideas.**

This variation in breastmilk is good, not bad. It means that breastmilk changes in response to the needs of the growing baby and his individual needs. But how have we turned this into something bad?

Breastmilk from a mother breastfeeding a baby of a certain age is not appropriate for a baby of another age

How absurd is that?

We receive emails, not uncommonly, asking, for example, if a mother can use breastmilk from her sister who is breastfeeding a ten month old. Her own baby

323

is only 3 months old and is not getting enough milk from her breast. "Would her sister's milk be okay for her 3 month old baby or should she supplement with formula instead?" Such questions come not only from mothers but also from lactation consultants. Doctors, with rare exceptions, do not ask, they just tell the mother it's not okay, without thinking about it. There are ways, incidentally, of **increasing the breastmilk production** of mother of the three month old, but this is discussed elsewhere in this book.

The question speaks volumes about the pernicious effectiveness of formula company marketing. However, let's think about this for just a minute. A given brand of formula doesn't change at all, assuming it was prepared according to directions. How is this better? If a baby requires different breastmilk at different ages or during the night compared to what he needs during the day, how does formula, which doesn't change at all, somehow become appropriate for babies of all ages? The formula "recommended" for a 2 day old, 2 week old, 2 month old is the same, *identical*. Formula, if we look at it biochemically, is **nothing like any breastmilk**, whether the breastmilk is from a mother breastfeeding a 2 day old, a 2 week old, a 2 month old, or a 2 year old. "Followup formulas" also called "follow on formulas" and "toddler formulas" which are almost completely unnecessary, do not get around this problem, as they are the same whether for a baby of 6 months or 12 months or 36 months.

Breastmilk sharing

Even pediatricians are ready to make absurd statements (not surprising as most have had nothing useful about breastfeeding in their training). Here is part of a statement from the Professional Association of Pediatricians with regard to breastmilk sharing (as reported in the Daily Mail October 17, 2012): "It (the Professional Association of Pediatricians in Germany) also warned that a newborn's nutritional needs differed from those of a baby even of several weeks or months old. The milk of a woman who already has an older child does not contain the right nutrient composition for a newborn, it added, and said women who were unable to breastfeed should use..." One is left perplexed and unable to comment at the absurdity of this statement. So, formula which does not change with time, is better for the baby than breastmilk which does change with time. The mind boggles.

Breastmilk banking

Many breastmilk banks will not accept milk from mothers breastfeeding a child older than 6 months, apparently for the same reasons as above. This is a terrible waste of potential donations, as it is often the mother who is breastfeeding a toddler who can most easily express milk for donation.

If there is no breastmilk available in the breastmilk bank, then a baby requiring supplementation would receive formula, and this is true whether the baby is a week old or 6 months old or premature. The same formula, chemically the same for all ages. How does this make sense?

It *doesn't* make sense. What does this tell us about how we view breastmilk and how we view formula? It says a lot. We believe that breastmilk is *intrinsically hazardous* while, at the same time, that formula is *intrinsically safe*. No matter how **different formula is from breastmilk**, we, as a society, as medical professional organizations, accept, somehow, that formula is superior to the breastmilk of a mother whose baby is of a different age than the possible recipient baby.

Of course, this can only be due to our love of and blind acceptance of "science", even if the "science" is actually formula company marketing and not based on science at all. See the formula company ad below, with all the meaningless lines to make the ad look scientific. It's an old ad, from the 1990s, when formula did not yet contain so many of the important ingredients the formula companies now tell us, indeed, warn us, are necessary for the baby's proper development, but apparently didn't need in the 1990s. And which now make **formula almost exactly like breastmilk** (even if formula does not change).

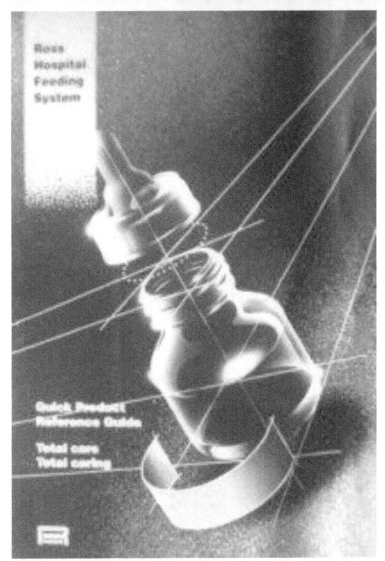

This ad for a formula published in the 1990s is trying to convince us that their formula is based on science. The lines on the ad have this intention, but in fact, are nothing but tangents to various circles. Meaningless.

HOW WHAT IS GOOD ABOUT BREASTFEEDING IS MADE BAD (PART 2)

Breastfeeding mothers and babies have a special relationship through the act of breastfeeding itself. Breastfeeding is much more than breastmilk, more than just another method of delivery of milk to the baby. Breastfeeding is a close physical and emotional relationship between two people who are usually very much in love with each other. This is not to say that mothers who bottle feed their babies do not love their babies. Only that the relationship of breastfeeding is *different* and special and good, good for the baby and the mother, good for the toddler and the mother. Even if the mother and baby are in skin to skin contact during a feeding, bottle feeding involves a baby's mouth in contact with an artificial material which feels nothing like the mother's breast to the baby and the bottle nipple, obviously, feels nothing. Breastfeeding involves the baby's very sensitive mucous membranes of the mouth in close and intimate contact with a very sensitive part of the mother's body. Surely everyone can understand this, though many do not.

Babies may want to go to the breast for many reasons. Not all of these reasons have to do with their being hungry. Even a young baby is usually comforted by the breast. The importance of the breastfeeding relationship is highlighted even more dramatically when the baby is older and goes to the breast to get comfort and re-assurance and yes, love. The older baby breastfeeds also as a way to fall asleep or go back to sleep at night, and wants to breastfeed when he hurts himself, is sick or is unhappy for any reason. Breastfeeding frequently helps and reassures the child in such situations when nothing else will.

Will breastfeeding in stressful or painful situations result in the child not being able to handle frustration? Some psychologists have suggested this. Oh please!! We all must learn to deal with frustration because frustration is a feature of modern life; it's not a reason to tell a mother, or a child, "no, you must learn to deal with frustration, you cannot have the breast".

The "physicality" of breastfeeding, as well as the ease with which breastfeeding can work when breastfeeding is free of "breastfeeding devices" is one reason that so many mothers want to get rid of the bottle or the **nipple shield**, even if the breastfeeding is "going well" with the nipple shield. As an aside, too often the nipple shield does *seem* to work for a while but may cause the milk **supply to decrease with time**, especially if the mother doesn't start out with an abundance of milk.

The "closeness" of breastfeeding is something that both mothers and babies cherish, and yet it may become a point of contention between mothers and physicians, especially, somewhat surprisingly, pediatricians. And also, between the mothers and their own families, all of whom may tell mothers that feeding the baby according to the baby's needs ("on demand" a phrase that speaks volumes how normal breastfeeding is perceived) causes the baby to be "spoiled", overly dependent, aggressively "needy", unable to "self-soothe" and, of course, "demanding".

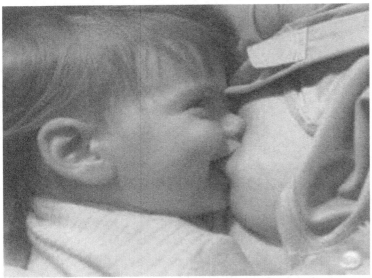

This twenty month old toddler loves to breastfeed, enjoys breastfeeding, and does not want to stop breastfeeding. He is breastfeeding for more than milk – he is breastfeeding because he loves to breastfeed.

These adjectives would not be used in tribal societies not yet exposed to "modern ideas", where babies are automatically breastfed, cuddled, held close and carried much of the time. See photo of a mother and baby in the Central African Republic. In industrial societies, the needs of the baby have more and more become subservient to the parents' needs and breastfeeding babies are required to be "efficient" and not impose on their parents.

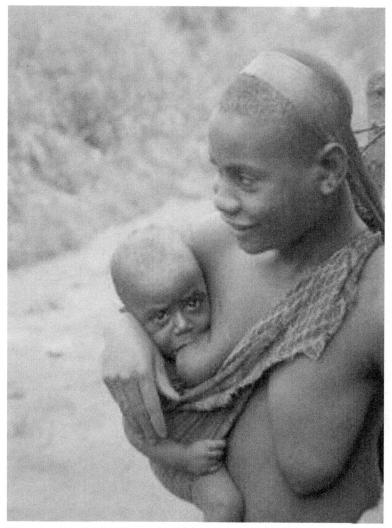

This mother in the Central African Republic lived, at the time I took this photo, in a society little touched by Western values. Babies were constantly carried, never refused the breast. And

fathers also spend a lot of time carrying the baby.

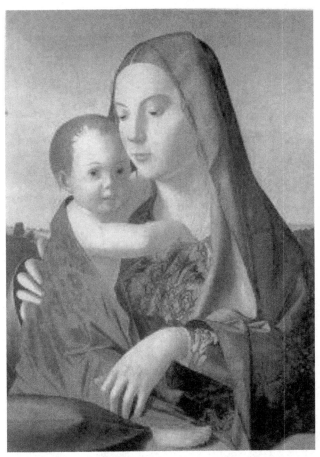

What does the baby's hand inside the mother's dress mean? Most mothers who are breastfeeding a toddler know. It means comfort and security for the baby.

One of the nicest aspects of breastfeeding is that it is an easy way to put babies to sleep; yet, mothers are also told not to let the baby fall asleep at the breast, to prevent the baby from "needing" the **breast to fall asleep**. Interestingly, I cannot remember a mother being told not to let the baby fall asleep while drinking from a bottle.

True, mothers *are* told not to let the baby sleep with the bottle in his mouth, as it may cause dental caries in the older baby, but they are not told to pull the bottle out of the baby's mouth just as the baby starts falling asleep on the bottle. Falling asleep on the breast is not "allowed" for the breastfeeding baby, however. Falling asleep while breastfeeding is seen as a prelude to "**sleep problems**". Falling asleep on the bottle is not seen as a prelude to "sleep problems", but rather "great, the baby fell asleep because he is full". Incidentally, breastfeeding the baby/toddler to sleep **does not cause dental caries** because of the complete difference between the way that bottle feeding works and how breastfeeding works. And how breastmilk is different from formula.

The notion that breastfeeding is merely just another delivery system for milk leads to other wrongheaded advice from health professionals. So, frequently mothers are told that a baby does not need to feed during the night by 6 to 9 months of age (some pediatricians will say even by 4 months of age), and the fact that your 7 month old baby is still waking up in the night means he has a **sleep problem** and needs "sleep training". How was it decided that a baby waking in the night is abnormal behaviour? Bottle feeding mentality! Bottle feeding formula often "stuffs" the baby at the "last" feeding of the day and so the baby sleeps longer. Bottle feeding parents are also more likely to "sleep train" their babies, which, essentially ignores the needs of the baby and teaches the baby to ignore his own needs.

The fact that the baby is likely waking up for the comfort and security of the breast and not necessarily for "food" (though sometimes for food) does not enter the mind of the pediatrician, physician, or public health nurse, etc. And once breastfeeding doesn't happen for "food" it becomes *dispensable, unnecessary, a waste of the mother's time*. The fact that breastfeeding is much more than a "natural" variety of bottle feeding, simply using a softer bottle, is something that is difficult for many, including health professionals, to integrate into their own bottle feeding way of thinking about infant feeding.

331

Parents are frequently told to ignore the emotional and other aspects of breastfeeding because the baby doesn't need them, the "adviser" completely unaware that these may actually take precedence over the "food" aspect of the needs of older babies. That older babies don't always perceive breastfeeding as food or drink can be seen when watching an older child breastfeed and ask for water or food in the middle of the breastfeed and then happily return to breastfeeding. All these good things breastfeeding provides are turned into negatives more and more as the baby grows older. So, a 2 year old falling asleep on the breast or wanting to breastfeed is seen as far more "dependent" than a young baby and a sign of the parents' failure to "train" the baby earlier on. In fact, the security of the breast results in a much more independent child and adult. A child does not become independent through insecurity; a child becomes independent when his need for security is assured and satisfied, by breastfeeding, amongst other things.

Mothers are blithely told very often that they must interrupt breastfeeding their toddler **because of medication the mother must take** and the fact that the toddler would cry day after day for hours at a time not being able to breastfeed is not even considered and the damage caused to the child seen as trivial. It is particularly galling because it is **almost never necessary to interrupt breastfeeding for medication**, even if the baby is a newborn.

Many mothers need to hear that it is fine (in fact it is not just fine, it is *normal*) to fulfill the needs of their baby or toddler and be reassured that breastfeeding is not just about fulfilling the baby's or toddler's need for milk. Most would be happy feeding the baby at night, would not mind feeding the baby whenever the baby desires etc. etc. but nevertheless are leaned on to feed the baby by the clock, or not put the baby to sleep at the breast, or stop night feedings. They are often humiliated and mocked by others for doing, essentially, what babies have throughout history come to expect.

Why is breastfeeding not always "ideal"?

Unfortunately, breastfeeding is not always ideal or as beautiful as suggested above, not by a long shot. Many problems arise for many mothers and babies,

332

most often because mothers are not getting started with breastfeeding in the ideal and beautiful way and not getting good help during those crucial first days or even after the first few days either. Mothers get **sore nipples, sore breasts,** the baby is **not getting enough from the breast** or the **mother is not getting the help** that she needs in order to get the **baby more milk** from the breast. Even something as simple, (simple, *if* the helper is experienced and skilled), as **how to latch a baby on** is rarely taught well. Mothers are burdened with "rules" on how to breastfeed, such as **"feed the baby on only one breast at a feeding"**, feed the baby by the clock, **use a nipple shield,** interrupt breastfeeding for **medications** all of which lead frequently to difficult breastfeeding.

In some countries, particularly the US, maternity leave is so inadequate, so pitiful, that breastfeeding often stops because the baby refuses the breast after being bottle fed much of the day, or the mother's milk supply decreases and cannot kept up with pumping.

And so many more ways breastfeeding is messed up for the mother and baby.

One example of how equating bottle feeding to breastfeeding causes problems for the mother and baby. From the article mentioned in the first line.

From a mother's email: "My baby was not gaining weight well, so the doctor suggested that I pump my milk and feed the baby by bottle so that we know how much he is getting."

There is **so much wrong** in this one sentence, which, unfortunately, is a frequent suggestion to mothers of babies not gaining well on breastfeeding alone!

This "suggestion" by the doctor implies that what a mother can pump is what the baby gets from the breast. This, from both clinical experience and more than **one study,** is clearly not true. A baby who is latched on well and breastfeeding well can get more than the mother can pump. A baby who is latched on poorly will usually not breastfeed well and thus get less from the

333

breast than the mother can pump. If the mother can pump as much as the baby needs for the baby to gain weight well, then the baby should be able to gain weight well by breastfeeding only. When dealing with breastfeeding issues, the mother and baby need *competent* help in order to get the baby breastfeeding well.

If, on the basis of this suggestion, the mother cannot pump or express all the milk the baby needs, the mother will be discouraged and may abandon breastfeeding altogether. Many mothers whose babies are gaining weight well breastfeeding exclusively cannot pump or express milk in sufficient quantities for the baby's requirements, even if the mother is separated from the baby for a day or two and pumps her milk regularly. Pumping or expressing tells us only about the mother's ability to pump or express; it has nothing do with breastfeeding, no matter how much some people try to identify pumping with breastfeeding.

Furthermore, the baby's "requirements" are based on what a formula fed, bottle fed baby would need and there is no evidence that quantities based on the formula fed baby's requirements apply to the exclusively breastfed baby's needs.

Even if there is breastmilk in the bottle, bottle feeding being a completely different feeding method and the flow from the bottle being constant implies that the baby will drink different quantities of milk than he would from the breast and would likely drink *too much*. Breastmilk is different and **studies** seem to show that between one and five months after birth, a mother's milk supply does not increase substantially. Breastmilk whose composition changes with time is different from formula that is constant in composition (if prepared properly) and thus, to make up for the inadequacy of formula, the formula fed baby's requirements increase with increasing weight.

What is most wrong about the advice given to the mother mentioned above is that too often the baby, after being on bottles for several days or longer, is likely to refuse to take the breast again. And that loss is a big loss, because breastfeeding is more than a method of delivering milk to a baby. Breastfeeding, actually *feeding the baby at the breast*, is both a physical and

334

emotional relationship, a close intimate physical and emotional relationship between two people who almost always love each other very much. Bottle feeding, even when there is breastmilk in the bottle, does not duplicate this relationship in any way.

See also the chapters **Breastfeeding a Toddler** and **The Right to Breastfeed**.

Made in the USA
Coppell, TX
11 June 2020

27456809R00184